Supreme Health and Fitness by Sean Ali!

PRESENTS:

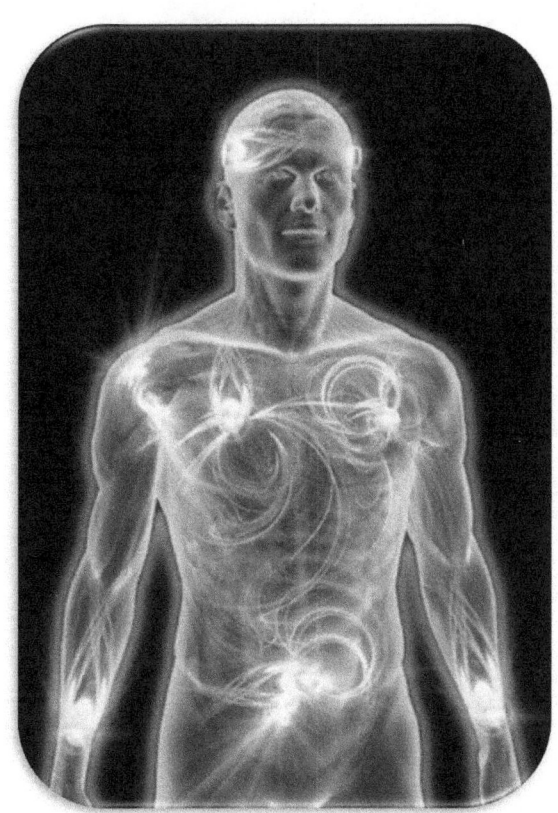

LIFE ENERGY !

THE SUN, GLUCOSE & WHY HUMANS ARE HERBIVORES!

Successfully Building and Maintaining Supreme Health and Fitness by Increasing the level of Knowledge and Science of Life!

Science Of Life Series * Volume 2

Supreme Health & Fitness by Sean Ali!

Achieving and Maintaining Supreme Health and Wellness by increasing the level of Knowledge and Science of Life!

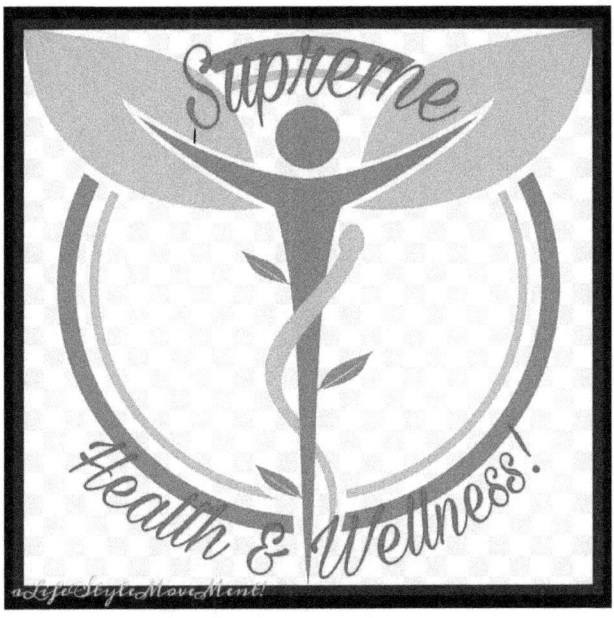

Assisting Scientist:

Khalil Malik * Kareem Tyree * Gabriella Monique

LIFE ENERGY !

THE SUN, GLUCOSE & WHY HUMANS ARE HERBIVORES!

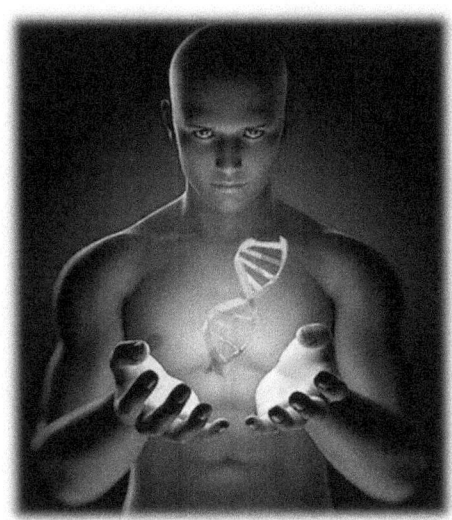

A Supreme Health and Fitness Production

*

Science Of Life ...... Volume 2

*

Achieving and Maintaining Supreme Health and Fitness by increasing the level of Knowledge and Science of Life!

SUPREME HEALTH & FITNESS

ENERGY AND NUTRITION IN HEALTH CARE

Nutrition and Health care has always been approached from the Physical Chemical properties of Us instead of focusing on and treating Us in from and Energy perspective.

A complete Comprehensive Energy Assessment will help provide the foundation for appropriate Energy Therapy based on identified Energy needs which in-turn allows one to successfully Build and Maintain your own Supreme Health and Fitness!

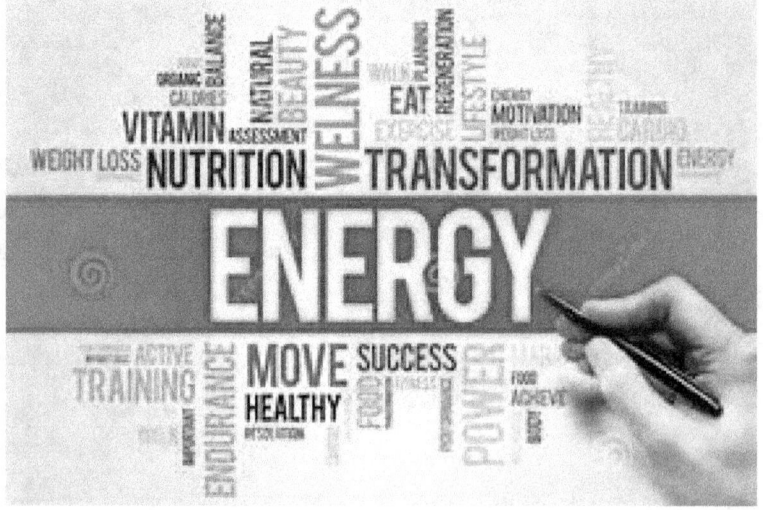

Table Of Contents

******

Introduction

*****

Peace and Blessings of Life!

In today's world, Nutrition is thought of as the Macro and Micro-Nutrients (Carbs, Vitamins, Mineral, Protein, Fat), but no one is living any longer since these discoveries and changing to eat according to this viewpoint of Nutrition.

The small book is presenting the understanding of Nutrition from an Energy specific, which equates Nutrition to the Quality and Quantity of Bio-available Life Energy. Everything in the Universe is comprised of Atoms, therefore regardless of the different ways it can be phrased, the by-product of the inter-action between more than on Atoms (Bonding) = Atomic Energy.

Searching for the best Health therapy for my Family, clients and self, led me to prioritizing what on us keeps us Alive and placing them in order of Importance. The Body is many Organs and Systems the operate in unison to create Us. Each Organ and System have their specific Energy/Nutritional needs.

When establishing Health and Fitness, the 1st System to be addressed is our Respiratory System and the 1st Organ to is our Lungs, which we address in Volume 1 of this Science Of Life Series. Oxygen deficiency causes pre-mature death at a faster rate than Nutritionally deficiency.

The next study was on how to treat the Whole Self without causing a deficiency or over-load in any System or Organ while doing so. This led me to go to the simplest form the we are made of – CELLS. We are basically trillions of Cells comprised to make the Molecules, that make the Tissues, that make the Organs that make Self.

OUR CELLS NEED OXYGEN AND GLUCOSE !!!!

OXYGEN IS THE BREATH OF LIFE IN ATOMIC FORM !!!!!

GLUCOSE IS THE SUN-LIGHT IN ATOMIC FORM !!!!!!!

THIS IS OUR LIFE ENERGY!

Researching with strict diets of the Naturally occurring foods that yield the highest Value and Quality of Glucose/Life Energy presented results where the Cells are not only able to maintain, but rejuvenate, causing a significant increase in Energy, Strength, and a noticeable Youthful Appearance !!!

So, the foundation of our Health and Fitness is built on the health of our Cells!

Nutritionally healthy and strong Cells = a Healthy and Strong Self !

Nutritional Quality and Value should then be based on the Quality and Value of the Atomic Energy available in the 'foods' we choose to consume. The Quality and Value is whether it's Negative or Positive Energy.

Our Primary source of Life Energy is manifested in the form of the Atomic Structure of GLUCOSE.

Glucose is the Sun's Energy in Atomic Form....which is why it plays a vital role from our Cells to our Brain Power and Function!

GLUCOSE IS A CARBOHYDRATE........THE ONLY SOURCE IS PLANTS !!!!

THERE IS NO LIFE ENERGY PRESENT IN ANY ANIMAL MEAT !!!!!!

Any 'Food' that we choose to eat will present Energy, the only difference is whether it's Negative/free-radical energy – or – Positive/Life Energy.

Animal meats, processed and manufactured food-like items, and even Vitamins, Minerals and Water DO NOT manifest any Life Energy !

Nutritional Health and Wellness is the equivalent of Life Energy Health!

We know that Life is Energy based, and death is a state that absent of Life Energy. So, this book is research into Life Energy, the Best Quality and Value, as well as proper application. Almost every dis-ease we suffer, from Cancers to colds and flus, bacterial infections and viruses, each of these dis-eases attack and disrupt our Life Energy on a Cellular level. So, having maximum Cellular Energy = Supreme Health and Fitness!

Our bodies are created to literally last Forever. In fact, they are continuously finding bones of human remains and they are carbon-dating into the millions of years.

The only thing is the Essence/Spirit is no longer present. Our Food choices is either the source of our pre-mature death, or the Foundation of Abundant LIFE !!!!!!

Eating according to our Anatomical structure and function is required for us to successfully manifest the Highest Quality of our Humanity, because at the root of Food lays the Principle that *You Are What You Eat.*

What we eat either takes away from our Humanity, or Building and helping to maintain Abundant LIFE !!!!!

This book is a Humble endeavor to present to you the best science and knowledge available to help us successfully Build and Maintain our own Supreme Health and Fitness and be able to enjoy the a full and active Life, while becoming qualified to Express and make Manifest the Highest Quality of Humanity = The Direct Express Image & Likeness of GOD !

Achieving and Maintaining Supreme Health and Fitness by Increasing the Level of Knowledge and Science of LIFE!

PEACE !

Sean Ali, Supreme Health and Fitness

The Sun is Most Common Source of Energy in Every Ecosystem

*The flow of energy in an ecosystem is an open system; **the sun** constantly gives the planet energy in the form of light while it is eventually used and lost in the form of heat throughout the trophic levels of a food web*

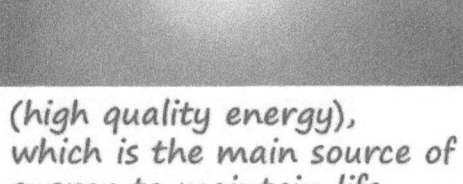

(high quality energy), which is the main source of energy to maintain life

*****

Chapter One ..... Role of Nutrition in Health Care!

*****

Nutrition Therapy plays an essential role in dis-ease management, and should always be at the fore-front of health care in general, and preventive health care specifically. Nutrition like all aspects of health is personal. For successful application, the way we approach Nutrition has to be re-examined and changed from a general, one-size-fits-all perspective, to the Realistic fact that Nutritional care must be approached from an individualistic concept.

BENEFITS OF NUTRITIONAL THERAPY

Improved health and well-being

Better sleep

Increased motivation and enthusiasm

Focused, quiet and alert mind

Loads of energy and stamina

Relief from unexplained pains, aches and itches

Younger skin, shinier hair and sparkling eyes

Improved digestion, circulation, and elimination

Stronger heart, lungs, tissues and bones

Reduced reactions to toxins and substances

Improved hormonal health and mental health

Prevention of cancer, candida, infections and many other health problems.

A Comprehensive Nutrition Assessment helps provide the necessary foundation for appropriate Nutrition

Therapy based on identified needs. Because Nutrition, like Health care, is personal, a Nutritional Assessment and Nutritional Therapy service promotes a main goal of assisting each individual in addressing their own specific Nutritional needs so they can HEAL themselves.

When we are suffering from a dis-ease, it is the direct result of an Energy imbalance within Self.

A Nutritional Assessment helps to pinpoint and address where and how we have an imbalance and Nutritional Therapy presents the adequate steps and foods to correct Self.

The role of Nutrition in health care is the equivalent of administering Bio-Medications. It enables us to make precise Energy adjustments through Nutrients to provide the proper Energy needed for any function/task – from Homeostasis, to regulations heart-beat, to exercising.

We come from the Earth and all our Solutions are manifested from the Earth. All we have to do is return back to the Earth and extract what we need. Food is that vehicle for administering the Life Energy in the form of Nutrition.

Food and the Energy released from it, presents as either the root cause of our dis-ease or the base for our Solution. From our Cells to our Immune system, we are Created to heal and regenerate Self through proper Nutrition. Our Food is our Medicine ONLY with proper application. There is no in-between, which means that we are either eating to die – OR – Eating To LIVE !!!!

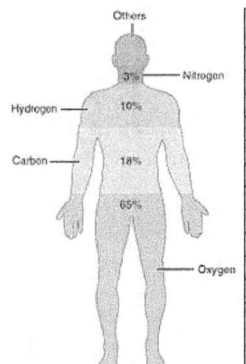

Element	Symbol	Percentage in Body
Oxygen	O	65.0
Carbon	C	18.5
Hydrogen	H	9.5
Nitrogen	N	3.2
Calcium	Ca	1.5
Phosphorus	P	1.0
Potassium	K	0.4
Sulfur	S	0.3
Sodium	Na	0.2
Chlorine	Cl	0.2
Magnesium	Mg	0.1
Trace elements include boron (B), chromium (Cr), cobalt (Co), copper (Cu), fluorine (F), iodine (I), iron (Fe), manganese (Mn), molybdenum (Mo), selenium (Se), silicon (Si), tin (Sn), vanadium (V), and zinc (Zn).		less than 1.0

Energy is the Key to LIFE and we now that the Sun is the Source of all Energy, then if we focus on how to obtain as much Sun as possible is the Key to Nutritional Health and Therapy.

We are comprised of Trillions of ATOMS. Atoms manifest Atomic Energy. This Atomic Energy is the foundation of our LIFE Energy. So our Health Care and Nutritional needs should be evaluated from an Atomic perspective. We should focus on the value and quality of Life/Atomic Energy.

Understanding and approaching our Health Care from an Energy perspective allows us to make Nutritional choices that provide the highest quality of Life/Atomic Energy = Successfully Building Supreme Health and Fitness!

During our childhood growth and development, our Food supplies the necessary Energy needed to unfold our DNA and make manifest the creation that is Us. After we are born, the same food now has the function of growth and development and maintaining our Creation.

One of the main benefits is helping to keep us here to enjoy a long and active Life, wherein we seemingly NEVER age!

The Quality of the food determines the value of Energy available for Growth, Development and Strength of our DNA and the determining factor in the overall Bond of our Atomic structure.

We are Naturally occurring Life forms and every part of Self can be referenced to specific parts of the Earth. For example, our Bones are as the Rocks on the Earth. Our Blood = the Water and our Skin/Tissue is related to the Vegetation.

Within the Chemical/Hydrogen Bonds that hold the Atoms of the Food together lies the LIFE ENERGY !!

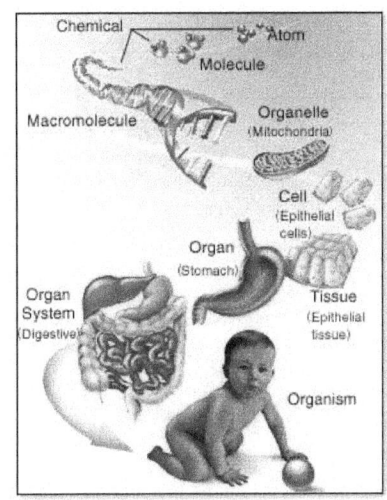

When we eat these Atomic structures, the act of Digestion Breaks these Bonds = Releasing the LIFE Energy !!!

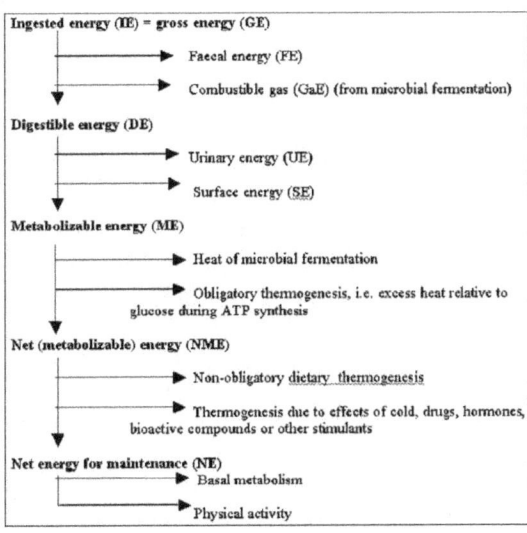

We know that Energy cannot be destroyed, but that it is transformed or transferred. The Life Energy that is within the Chemical Composition of Fruits and Veggies, is released during Digestion and Transferred to our Cells to provide Life for us as it was for the Plants.

From a simplified equation, we are a sack of water with chemicals in a solution. How these chemicals interact determines what we are to be, but in many of the interactions these Chemicals are used up or altered and must be replenished.

Nutrition consists of the proper consumption and assimilation of foods containing those necessary Chemicals.

Because only a few foods contain all or most of our needed Nutrients, we have to obtain them in a variety of foods. Within the last 50 years as people have moved further from quality food sources, while simultaneously food companies have changed the foods grown to have longer shelf life, our diets have changed dramatically. For about the last 100 years we have been bombarded with food-like products that are high in the negative values of synthetic chemicals, refined foods, sugar, and salt which have replaced many of the naturally occurring foods that our Ancestors ate.

The TOXIC Refined Simple Sugars so dominate our lives that they have become ubiquitous, present even in common table salt. Here in the United States, approximately 100 years ago, we consumed 3 Pounds of sugar per person per year; we now consume ***140 to 180 POUNDS***. This excessively high consumption of this TOXIC product plays a major role in one of the most devastating diseases—Obesity.

The federal government has stepped in to encourage some nutritional changes, which includes the following: (1) dramatic cutbacks in sugar and salt consumption, (2) increased consumption of foods containing Fiber, and (3) vast decrease in consumption ofMmilk products and other animal fat products. I would expand on this to say: eat ONLY naturally occurring Whole Grains, fresh Fruit, and Veggies and, IF you eat any animal meats, eat mostly fish.

Three facts about matter:

1. Atoms last forever
2. Atoms make up the mass of all materials.
3. Atoms are bonded to other atoms in molecules.

Two facts about energy:

1. Energy lasts forever. Energy is never created or destroyed in chemical changes.
2. Energy can be transformed from one form to another. Some common forms of energy include:
   - Heat
   - Light
   - Motion
   - Chemical energy: energy stored in bonds of molecules

How Crops Are Genetically Modified

Traditional Breeding	Mutagenesis	RNA Interference	Transgenics
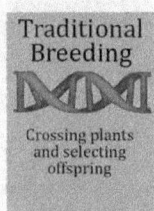	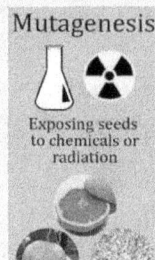	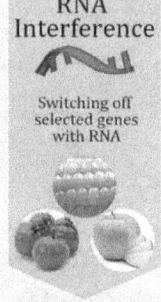	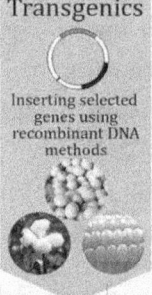
Crossing plants and selecting offspring	Exposing seeds to chemicals or radiation	Switching off selected genes with RNA	Inserting selected genes using recombinant DNA methods

Almost All Crops

Number of Genes Affected

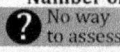

10K - >300K	No way to assess	1- 2	1 - 4
Desired gene(s) inserted with other genetic material. No safety testing requirements.	Random changes in genome, usually unpredictable. No safety testing requirements.	Targeted gene(s) switched off or 'silenced'. Safety testing required.	Desired gene(s) inserted only at known locations. Safety testing required.

*****

Chapter Two .... Genetically Modified Foods!

*****

Genetically Modified Organisms (GMO) are plants or bacteria in which the natural DNA has been changed/altered/grafted in some way to produce a specific and/or desired trait. Genetic modification can take place through plant breeding methods or through bio-technology in which a Gene is transferred from one organism to another. Genetic engineering was first applied in the pharmaceutical industry, and GMO bacteria produce human insulin for managing diabetes.

GMO food crops were introduced in the early 1990s, and their use has grown dramatically. Farmers in at least countries are planting GM species, representing 51% of the soybeans, 31% of the maize, and 5% of the rapeseed (canola oil) produced worldwide. In the United States, the sale and use of GM seeds are regulated by the *Food and Drug Administration* (FDA), the *Environmental Protection Agency* (EPA), and the *USDA*.

Goals for Genetic Modification

Since we humans first began to cultivate plants and populations have significantly increased, various practices have been used to improve the yield or desirability of particular species. Scientists begin to become involved in Agriculture and growing food became a scientific experiment. They begin using Mendel's principles of inheritance which introduced the development of hybrid plants and led to the 'Green revolution' , as well as new varieties of Wheat and Rice, that were able to presen double the yields. Such advances were credited with reducing food shortages in the developing world – *BUT NOT IN IMPROVING THE QUALITY AND VALUE OF LIFE.*

Genetic modification of food plants has three goals:

1. *Resistance to insects and disease:* Plants carrying a protein that acts as a built-in insecticide enable farmers to reduce their use of pesticides and herbicides.

2. *Increased tolerance to weather conditions:* Varieties able to survive more extreme environmental conditions are less likely to be destroyed by a late frost.

3. *Increased nutritional value:* Genetic modification increased the monounsaturated fatty acid content of soybean oil, and scientists are working on a tomato with increased amounts of lycopene. Grains with increased protein or micronutrients lessen nutrient deficiencies in developing nations.

Corn, Soybeans, Rapeseed (canola oil), Papaya, and Squash are among the genetically altered food crops approved for use in the United States.

Safety of Genetically Modified Crops

Both scientists and consumers have voiced concerns about GM foods as follows:

• *Risk of allergic reaction:* Transfer of a known allergen into a new food (for example: adding a peanut allergen to a corn plant) would make the modified plant unsafe for persons with the allergy.

• *Potential toxicity:* Need to check DNA against a Protein database to identify any known harmful Protein.

• *Danger to the environment:* Transfer of insect-resistant genes to weeds or invasive plants could be harmful to helpful insects such as butterflies. Farmers are urged to confine GM plants to specific growing areas because of the run-off into the surround earth which makes the ground TOXIC.

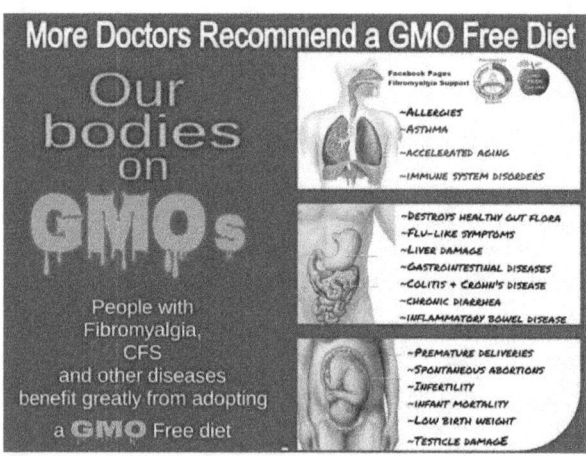

Current labeling regulations do not require the identification of ingredients from GM sources unless the modification has increased its Allergenicity or reduced its Nutrient content.

This situation is controversial as many consumers wish to avoid eating any Toxic GM foods. A requirement that a GM food carry label identification would provide the information needed for making an informed decision. GMO, Processed and/or manufactured food-like items manifest an Un-Natural Energy, that due to HOW it is made, when eaten, it releases TOXIC Energy when we attempt to Digest it.

Naturally occurring Fruits and Veggies manifest and release Natural Life Energy, that when we Digest = Supreme Health and Fitness.

Our environment here in America, is one which promotes the consumption of **Energy-Dense** food-like items, while providing limited need or opportunity for the expenditure of the Energy gained from these food-like products, has been referred to as "OBESOGENIC," and is the root cause to the ever increasing Obesity problem.

Put this in contrast to earlier times when humans survived as "hunter-gatherers," we now have a plentiful supply of good-tasting, high-calorie food, with little physical activity required to obtain it. The ever-present vending machine, special offers of two hamburgers for the price of one, and accessible food at all sporting and most social events all contribute to excessive food intake.

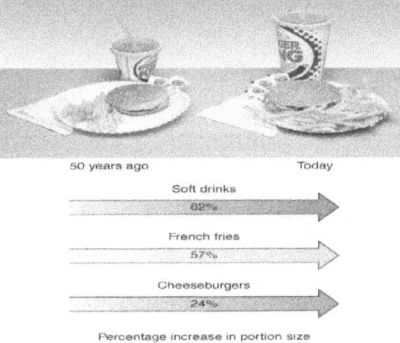

50 years ago   Today

Soft drinks
62%

French fries
57%

Cheeseburgers
24%

Percentage increase in portion size

Add to this the trend of portions served at fast-food restaurants being two to five times larger than those offered 20 years ago, and food served at home often equals three to four times the serving size referred to in meal planning guides.

Most people increase their energy intake when more food is served, adding to the potential for overeating at "all you can eat" food outlets.

Nutritional Assessment Form

Name: _____ ID: _____ Date: _____

1. How many meals and snacks to you eat each day? Meals _____ Snacks _____
   What type of snacks do you eat? _____

2. How many times a week to you eat the following meals away from home?
   Breakfast _____ Lunch _____ Dinner _____

3. What types of eating places do you frequently visit? (Check all that apply)
   Fast-Food _____ Diner/cafeteria _____ Restaurant _____ Other _____
   Starbucks/Coffee shop _____ Donut Shop _____

4. On average, how many pieces of fruit or glasses of juice do you eat or drink daily?
   Fresh fruit _____ Juice (8-oz cup) _____

5. On average, how many servings of vegetables do you eat each day? _____

6. How many times a week do you eat red meat? _____

7. How many times a week do you eat chicken or turkey? _____

8. How many time a week do you eat fish or shellfish? _____

9. How many hours of TV do you watch each day? _____

10. Do you usually snack while watching TV? Yes _____ No _____

11. How many times a week do you eat desserts and sweets? _____

12. How many servings of each of these drinks do you consume daily?

Water _____	Milk:	Alcohol:
Juice _____	Whole milk _____	Beer _____
Soda _____	2% milk _____	Wine _____
Diet soda _____	1% milk _____	Hard liquor _____
Sports drinks _____	Skim milk _____	
Iced tea _____		
Iced tea with sugar _____		

13. How many days per week do you do at least 30 minutes of continuous exercise (walking, biking, swimming, resistance training, health club, etc). _____

14. Exercise
    a) How many days a week do you exercise? _____
    b) How long does your workout last? _____
    c) What type (s) of exercise do you do?
    _____

Approximate daily caloric requirements for weight maintenance _____

Approximate daily calories patient is currently consuming _____

Approximate daily caloric expenditure from exercise _____

Excess calories patient is currently consuming _____

Dietary Reference Intake Values for Energy: Estimated Energy Requirement (EER) Equations and Values for Active Individuals by Life Stage Group

Life Stage Group	EER Prediction Equation	EER for Active Physical Activity Level (kCal\day)[a]	
		Male	Female
0–3 mo	EER = (89 × weight of infant in kg − 100) + 175	538	493 (2 mo)[c]
4–6 mo	EER = (89 × weight of infant in kg − 100) + 56	606	543 (5 mo)[c]
7–12 mo	EER = (89 × weight of infant in kg − 100) + 22	743	676 (9 mo)[c]
1–2 y	EER = (89 × weight of infant in kg − 100) + 20	1046	992 (2 y)[c]
3–8 y			
Male	EER = 88.5 − (61.9 × Age in yrs) + PA[b][(26.7 × Weight in kg) + (903 × Height in m)] + 20	1742 (6 y)[c]	
Female	EER = 135.3 − (30.8 × Age in yrs) + PA[b][(10.0 × Weight in kg) + (934 × Height in m)] + 20		1642 (6 y)[c]
9–13 y			
Male	EER = 88.5 − (61.9 × Age in yrs) +PA[b][(26.7 × Weight in kg) + (903 × Height in m)]+ 25	2279 (11 y)[c]	
Female	EER = 135.3 − (30.8 × Age in yrs) + PA[b][(10.0 × Weight in kg) + (934 × Height in m)] + 25		2071(11 y)[c]
14–18 y			
Male	EER = 88.5 − (61.9 − Age in yrs) + PA[b][(26.7 × Weight in kg) + (903 × Height in m)]+ 25	3152 (16 y)[c]	
Female	EER = 135.3 − (30.8 × Age in yrs) + PA[b][(10.0 × Weight in kg) + (934 × Height in m)] + 25		2368 (16 y)[c]
19 and older			
Males	EER = 662 − (9.53 × Age in yrs) +PA[b][(15.91 × Weight in kg) + (539.6 × Height in m)]	3067 (19 y)[c]	
Females	EER = 354 − (6.91 × Age in yrs) + PA[b][(9.36 × Weight in kg) + (726 × Height in m)]		2403 (19 y)[c]
Pregnancy			
14–18 y			
1st trimester	Adolescent EER + 0		2368 (16 y)[c]
2nd trimester	Adolescent EER + 340		2708 (16 y)[c]
3rd trimester	Adolescent EER + 452		2820 (16 y)[c]
19–50 y			
1st trimester	Adult EER + 0		2403 (19 y)[c]
2nd trimester	Adult EER + 340		2743 (19 y)[c]
3rd trimester	Adult EER + 452		2855 (19 y)[c]
Lactation			
14–18 y			
1st 6 mo	Adolescent EER + 330		2698 (16 y)[c]
2nd 6 mo	Adolescent EER + 400		2768 (16 y)[c]
19–50 y			
1st 6 mo	Adult EER + 330		2733 (19 y)[c]
2nd 6 mo	Adult EER + 400		2803 (19 y)[c]

[a] The intake that meets the average energy expenditure of active individuals at a reference height, weight, and age.

[b] See table entitle "Physical Activity Coefficients (PA Values) for Use in EER Equations" to determine the PA value for various ages, genders, and activity levels.

[c] Value is calculated for an individual at the age in parentheses.

*****

Chapter Three .... Nutritional and Energy Status!

*****

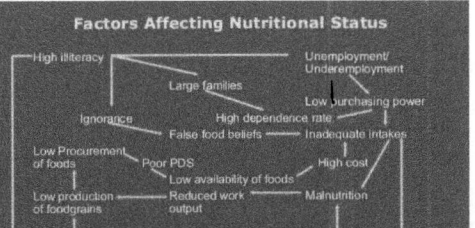

The Nutritional and Energy Status of each individual can be established by Measuring Indicators of our Nutrient Stores.

Nutrient Stores (Table 2.1) refers to the storage capacity in our Bodies of Life Energy.

Nutrient Status refers to the amount of Life Energy available.

Nutrients are the classification of Life Energy manifested from the 'Breaking" of the Atomic Bonds in our food during Digestion.

Food Energy is the Atomic/Chemical Energy that we receive our food. Along with Molecular Oxygen and through the process of Cellular Respiration, our food is converted into Energy.

Cellular Respiration is the Physiological act that involves either the process of joining Oxygen from Air with the Molecules of food = Aerobic Respiration; or the process of reorganizing the Atoms within the Molecules = Anaerobic Respiration.

This process means that variations of our Nutrient Stores result in immediate and simultaneous changes in our Nutritional Status. This manifests when our Nutrient Needs and Nutrient Use are increased or alterations in Nutrient Intake occur. Examples would be during fasting, binge eating or fad dieting.

TABLE 2.1   Estimated Energy Stores in Humans

Energy source	Storage site	Approximate energy (kcal)
ATP/CP*	Various tissues	5
Carbohydrate	Blood glucose	80
	Liver glycogen	400
	Muscle glycogen	1,500
Fat	Serum free fatty acids	7
	Serum triglycerides	75
	Muscle triglycerides	2,500
	Adipose tissue	80,000+
Protein	Muscle protein	30,000

*ATP/CP = adenosine triphosphate/creatine phosphate

Any presentation of an inadequacy, deficiency or excess of a particular Nutrient produces an equivalent Physiologic alteration in the Energy available for our Body.

Naturally occurring Plants (Fruits, Veggies, Grains) provide Natural Life Energy, that when eaten, Strengthens, Heals and Maintains our Physical Bodies and helping to Balance and Focus our Mental and Spiritual.

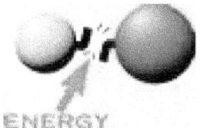

ENERGY

Everything Is ATOMS – INCLUDING NUTRIENTS !

Energy and human life

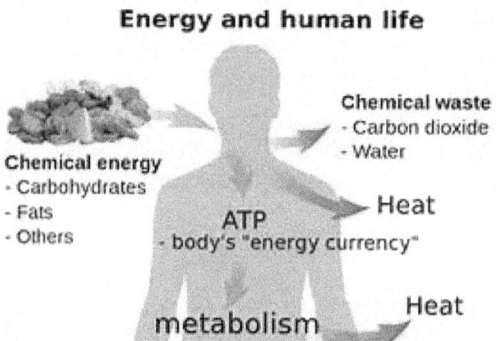

It is the TOXIC Energy that is a by-product of the Chemical Bonds of the processed/manufactured food-like items, which releases Free-Radical Energy, that Causes a negative disruption in our Energy balance and health.

This reaction is at the root cause of dis-eases, sicknesses and pre-mature death (BAD Atomic re-actions).

Each food item has a specific Metabolizable Energy Intake (MEI). This value can be approximated by Multiplying the total amount of Energy associated with a food item by 85%, which is the typical amount of Energy that is actually obtained by us after Cellular Respiration has been accomplished.

Fats and Ethanol (Alcohol) have the highest available amount of food Energy per mass, 37 and 29 kJ/g (9 and 7 KCal/g), respectively. Proteins and most Carbohydrates have about 17 kJ/g (4 kcal/g).

The differing Energy Density of foods (Fat, Alcohols, Carbohydrates and Proteins) lies mainly in their varying proportions of Carbon, Hydrogen, and Oxygen Atoms. Their specific arrangements determines the quality and value of their respective Bio-available Energy.

Carbohydrates have an Atomic arrangement that manifests the preferred Life Energy for our Growth and Development.

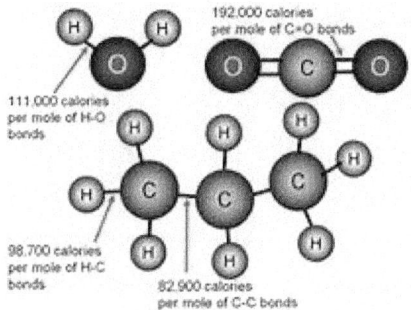

These combinations determine How and If or bodies need these Energies, also when and the amount. From this Atomic formula, Carbohydrates are the Primary source of Life Energy.

Carbohydrates that are not easily absorbed, such as Fiber, or Lactose in lactose-intolerant individuals, contribute less food Energy.

The amount of Water, Fat, and Fiber in foods determines those foods' specific Energy density.

Chloroplasts, Mitochondria, and the Energy Cycle

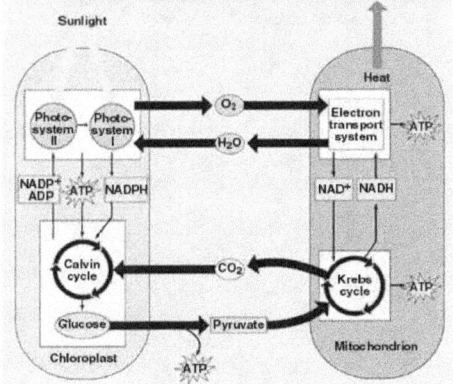

Bio- molecules

Life ←   → **Two or more atoms
bonded together**

- **Bio-molecules** are large molecules that make up living things.

Carbohydrates
(sugars)

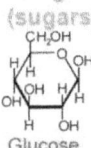
Glucose

Proteins

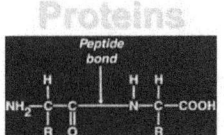

Nucleic Acids

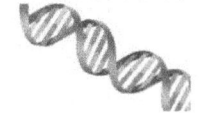

Lipids (fats)

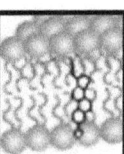

*****

Chapter Four .... The Science of Nutrition!

*****

Nutrition builds on two primary areas of Science - The Life Sciences of Bio-Chemistry and Physiology, which tells us how Nutrition relates to our physical health and body function. The Behavioral Sciences help us understand how Nutrition is interwoven with our Psychosocial needs. Both aspects are simultaneously and constantly at work in our lives.

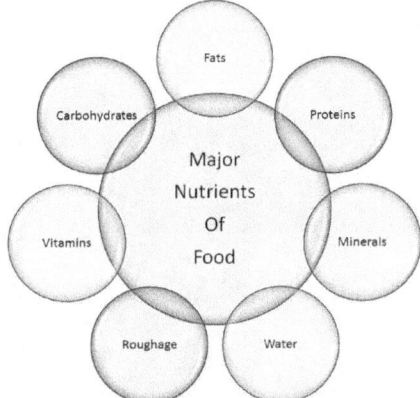

Human Organisms are highly complex groupings of Chemical compounds constantly at work in an array of reactions that sustain life. Nutrients provide the needed Life Energy to participate in and help control these Chemical reactions.

Various Physiologic systems integrate the activities of millions of functioning Cells, uniting them into a functioning Whole = Self. This highly sensitive internal control is called **Homeostasis**.

We also have social and emotional qualities rooted in our earliest awareness. Eating patterns and attitudes toward food develop over a lifetime based on the influences of our primary family and friends, ethnic or cultural group, community, nation, and world.

How we perceive food, what we choose to eat, why we eat what we do, and the ways in which we eat are all integral to human nutrition.

Nutrition, which means *to Nourish*, encompasses the food people eat and how it enriches their lives physically, socially, and personally. From the moment of conception until death, an appropriate supply of food provides the necessary Life Energy that facilitates and supports optimal growth and maturation of both our Mental and Physical well-being.

Good nutrition promotes health and reduces the risk of adverse conditions ranging from low birth weight to obesity to cardiovascular disease. Food supplies the Energy to carry out our body functions, such as Inhaling and Exhaling (Respiration), maintaining consistent 98.6° Body temperature, and engaging in and completing physical activity.

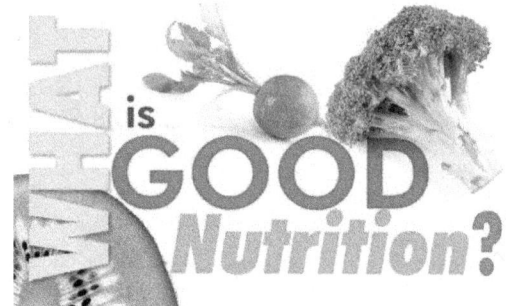

Food also nourishes the Human Spirit. We all have our particular "soul foods," comfort foods that connect us to our family and provide a sense of Psychological and emotional well-being.

To complete the study of Nutrition, we need to also define the terms that describe this body of Knowledge and the health professionals who work within it.

Nutrition refers to the food people eat and how it nourishes their bodies.

Nutrition Science defines the Nutrient requirements for our body maintenance, growth, activity, and reproduction.

Dietetics is the health profession with primary responsibility for the practical application of nutrition science throughout the life cycle in health and disease.

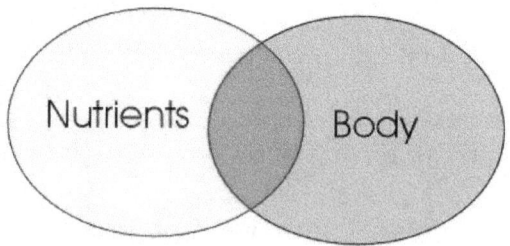

The Scope Nutritional Science

Nutrients

Body

The **Registered Dietitian (RD) or Registered Dietitian Nutritionist (RDN)** is the nutrition expert on the health care team, and in collaboration with the physician and nurse, carries the major responsibility for a patient's nutritional care.

Public Health Nutritionists focus on disease prevention and oversee programs that serve high-risk groups in the community such as pregnant teens or older adults, assessing needs, and applying interventions. RDs cooperate with school nurses to teach weight-management classes for children and parents, assist day care providers in planning menus and snacks, or help clients at fitness centers improve their body composition or athletic performance.

For more than a century, the U.S. Department of Agriculture (USDA) has been trying to improve our eating habits by issuing dietary recommendations. It currently spends $333.3 million per year educating the public about what we should and should not consume and in what quantities (USDA, 1997). That seems a great expenditure until we consider that America's food manufacturers spend that amount promoting snacks and nuts; their total annual advertising budget is more than $7 billion, most of which is spent promoting highly processed, packaged foods.

The fast-paced American lifestyle relies on these convenience foods and on restaurant and take-out fare. We now spend 45% of our food dollars on away-from-home meals and snacks, most of which are higher in fat, salt, and sugar and lower in fiber and calcium than meals prepared at home.

According to the USDA's Healthy Eating Index, some small improvements have been made in the American diet. On a scale of 1 to 100, the average U.S. score rose from 61.5 in 1990 to 63.8 in 1995, but it still falls far short of the 80 or above that marks a good diet. Put another way, Americans are earning about a C− in healthy eating practices.

Nutritionists, physicians, research scientists, alternative practitioners, food manufacturers, and consumers hold differing views about what percentage of calories we should obtain from each macronutrient.

People favoring a largely vegetarian, low-fat diet tend to recommend that we receive about 15% of our calories from protein, 60% from carbohydrates, and 25% from fats.

Proponents of high-protein diets often advocate 30% protein, 40% carbohydrates, and 30% fats.

Although these numbers may provide useful guidelines, they do not address one crucial factor: the QUALITY of the Nutrients in each category.

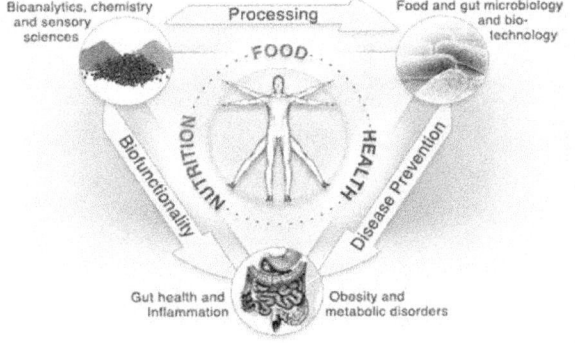

The food pyramid, which recommends 6 to 11 servings of grain-based foods, fails to distinguish, for example, between the empty calories of frozen waffles, which are composed primarily of white sugar and white flour, and a bowl of whole-grain cereal.

It encourages us to use fats "sparingly" but advocates 2 or 3 helpings of cheese and whole milk, which contain at least 8 g of fat per serving, plus up to 3 servings of meat, which can contain up to 26 Grams of Fat per serving. It also doesn't differentiate between processed/un-natural Fats that are TOXIC versus the naturally occurring Healthy Fats that we Need.

Is a Whopper (40 g of fat) part of a healthy diet?

Are PopTarts (20 g of white sugar) giving us the right kind of energy to start the day?

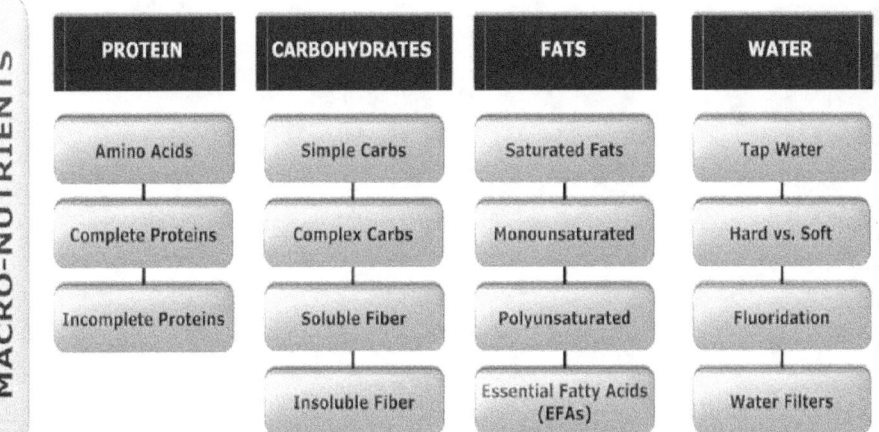

*****

Chapter Five .... Functions of Food and Nutrients!

*****

Food serves as the vehicle for bringing **Nutrients** into the body; and these specific Chemical Compounds and Elements in food—the nutrients—are the substances that manifest the Energy our body needs.

No one particular food or food combination is required to ensure health. The human race has survived for centuries on a wide variety of foods, depending on what was available and what the culture designated as appropriate.

There are Approximately 50 Nutrients that are known to be Essential to human life and health. Countless other elements and molecules are being studied and may be found to be essential.

Pyramid of Energy

Tertiary consumer 10 kcal

Secondary consumer 100 kcl

Primary consumer 1000 kcal

Producers 10,000 kcal

Decreasing rate of energy flow

The identification of **Essential Nutrients** is especially important when developing a comprehensive Energy dense dietary plan.

The Essential Nutrients include the **Macro-Nutrients (Carbohydrates, Fats, and Proteins)**, the **Micro-Nutrients** (Vitamins and Minerals), and water. The Macronutrients supply our Life Energy and Build Tissue, whereas the Micronutrients, needed in much smaller amounts, form specialized structures and regulate our Body processes.

Water is the additional and often-forgotten Nutrient that sustains all of our Life Systems. The sum of all the Chemical Reactions occurring in our body that use Nutrients is referred to as **Metabolism**.

Nutrients have three general functions, as follows:

1. To provide Energy

2. To build and repair body tissues and structures

3. To regulate the metabolic processes that maintain homeostasis.

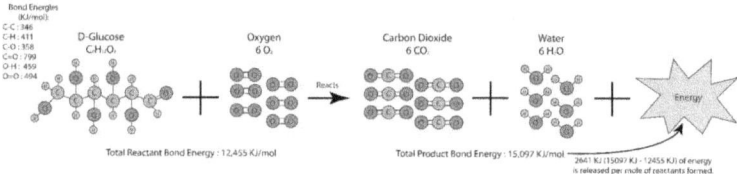

Energy

All three of the macronutrients—carbohydrate, fat, and protein—can be used for the production of Kcals Energy, although Carbohydrates, particularly in the form of Glucose, is our Life Energy source.

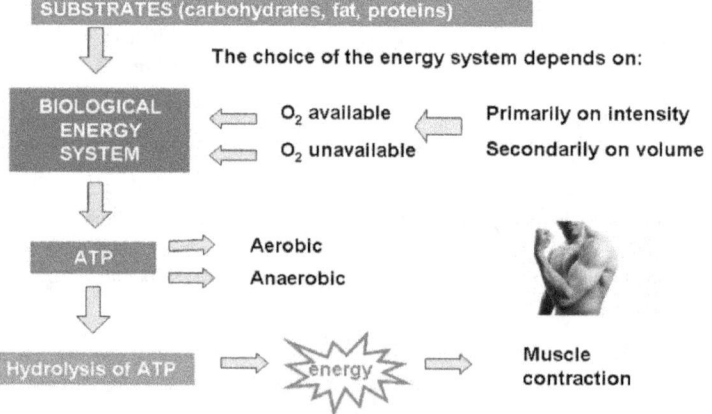

Tissue Building and Repair

Protein is the primary nutrient for building and maintaining body tissues. Vitamins and minerals are used in smaller amounts in the structure of specialized tissues.

Protein.

Proteins are broken down into **amino acids,** the building blocks for body growth and repair. Body tissues are constantly being broken down and rebuilt to ensure growth and maintenance of body structure. Proteins also form vital substances such as enzymes and hormones that regulate body systems.

Minerals.

Minerals help build tissues with very specific functions. The major minerals—calcium and phosphorus—give strength to bones and teeth. The trace element iron is a component of hemoglobin and binds oxygen for transport to cells and carbon dioxide for return to the lungs. Minerals serve as cofactors in controlling cell metabolism. One example is iron, which controls the enzyme actions in the cell mitochondria that produce and store high-energy compounds.

Vitamins.

Vitamins are complex molecules needed in very minute amounts but are essential in certain tissues. Vitamin C produces the intercellular ground substance that cements tissues together and prevents tissue bleeding. Vitamin A in the rods and cones of the eye is needed for vision in dim light. Many vitamins are components of cell enzyme systems. They govern reactions that produce energy and **synthesize** important molecules. For example, thiamin controls the release of energy for cell work and vitamin B_{12} is needed for the synthesis and maturation of red blood cells.

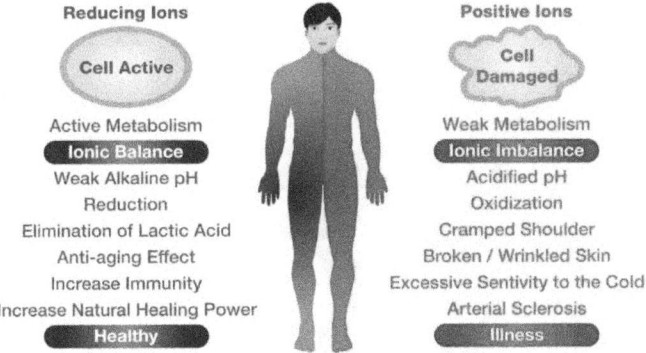

Reducing Ions	Positive Ions
Cell Active	**Cell Damaged**
Active Metabolism	Weak Metabolism
Ionic Balance	**Ionic Imbalance**
Weak Alkaline pH	Acidified pH
Reduction	Oxidization
Elimination of Lactic Acid	Cramped Shoulder
Anti-aging Effect	Broken / Wrinkled Skin
Increase Immunity	Excessive Sentivity to the Cold
Increase Natural Healing Power	Arterial Sclerosis
Healthy	**Illness**

Metabolic Regulation

Specific vitamins and minerals are necessary for enzyme activities responsible for a host of chemical reactions. Water provides the appropriate environment for these reactions to occur.

Water.

Water forms the blood, lymph, and intercellular fluids that transport nutrients to cells and remove waste. Water also functions as a regulatory agent, providing the fluid environment in which all metabolic reactions take place.

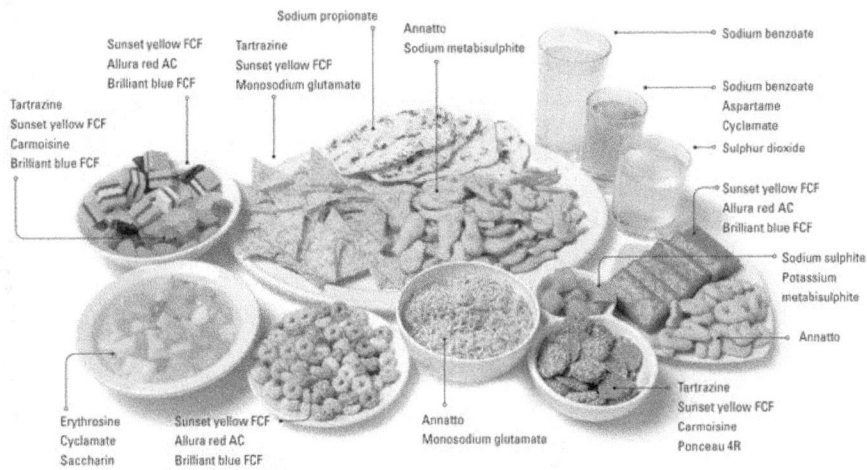

*****

Chapter Six …. Modern Nutrition: REPLACING MOTHER NATURE

*****

Fast-forwarding to the twentieth century, we find a very different picture of food production and consumption. Early in the century, advances in biochemistry allowed scientists to isolate some of the active ingredients in food. In 1928, for example, it was discovered that limes, the British Navy's traditional method of preventing scurvy, worked by providing sailors with vitamin C. Unfortunately, although vitamin C supplements proved easier to store and dispense, they did not provide the full benefits of the fruit. Later research disclosed that lime pulp contains *bioflavonoids,* which are necessary for absorbing and processing vitamin C. Bioflavonoids also help maintain collagen and capillary walls and protect against infection and cancer. Scientists were discovering that replacing natural products with artificial ones did not always improve on the original.

A CLOSER LOOK AT SUGAR SUBSTITUTES

Sweetener	Brand or Trade Names	Number of Times as Sweet as Table Sugar	Natural or Artificial, Caloric Content	Other Notable Effects
Saccharin	Sweet 'N Low, Sweet Twin, Necta Sweet	200 – 700	Artificial – no calorie	
Aspartame	Nutrasweet, Equal, Sugar Twin	160 – 220	Artificial – no calorie	In people with the rare genetic condition phenylketonuria, aspartame cannot be properly processed by the body and therefore it must carry FDA warning label
Acesulfame K	Sunett, Sweet & Safe, Sweet One	200	Artificial – no calorie	
Sucralose	Splenda	600	Artificial – no calorie	Suitable for cooking and baking
Neotame	Neotame	8000	Artificial – no calorie	Sweetening not reduced by heating
Rebaudioside A	Enliten, PureVia, Stevia, Sun Crystals, SweetLeaf	40 – 300	Natural plant extract (Stevia), also manufactured artificially – no calorie	
Stevia/Erythritol	Truvia	300	Natural – no calorie	
Sorbitol	Sorbitol	0.5 – 0.7	Natural polyol found in apples, pears, peaches, and prunes Can be man-made – low calorie	Laxative effect if recommended dose exceeded
Mannitol	Mannitol	0.5 – 0.7	Natural polyol found in a wide variety of foods, including almost all plants Can be man-made – low calorie	Laxative effect if recommended dose exceeded
Xylitol	Xylitol	1	Natural polyol occurring in many fruits and vegetables Can be man-made – low calorie	Has natural anti-tooth-decay properties Laxative effect if recommended dose exceeded

This finding, however, did not stop scientists from trying to improve on nature. Currently, modern technology and agribusiness have "improved" crops by covering them with artificial chemicals, including pesticides, fungicides, ripening agents, and fumigants, all of which make them more efficient to grow, ship, and store. Genetic engineering has changed the biological structure of many plants in ways not yet fully understood. Some plants are irradiated (flooded with "harmless" radiation) to lengthen their shelf life. Animals destined for the table are dosed with antibiotics to prevent disease and with hormones to make them fat and juicy.

Once vegetables, fruit, milk, meat, and eggs leave the farm, they are often "processed" into "food products," such as canned soup and frozen dinners. Processed foods are generally high in fat, salt, and sugar; are lower in nutrients than fresh foods; and contain a host of chemicals to boost flavor, color, texture, and shelf life. Consider the following:

- Pounds of sugar the average American consumed per year in the nineteenth century: less than 10

- Pounds of sugar the average American consumes per year today: 150

ARTIFICIAL SWEETENER TOXICITY

DO YOU DRINK DIET SODA + ENERGY DRINKS?

HEADACHES	MIGRAINES
INCREASED APPETITE	HYPERACTIVITY
BLURRED VISION	INTESTINAL IMBALANCE
MEMORY LOSS	DIZZINESS
ANXIETY	INSOMNIA
SWELLING	JOINT PAIN
NAUSEA	MILD DEPRESSION
MENSTRUAL IRREGULARITY	HEART ARRHYTHMIA

Jennifer Leigh
Medical Nutrition

Among the many artificial substances used in processed foods are such synthetic sweeteners as aspartame, silicon dioxide, phenylalanine, tribasic calcium phosphate, benzosulfimide, and calcium silicate.

The effects of all these chemicals on our bodies are not entirely known, but saccharin, the first widely used artificial sweetener, was shown to cause cancer in laboratory animals.

Aspartame (NutraSweet) is now being studied for possible neurological effects. Large quantities of one of its ingredients, methanol, have been shown to cause blindness, brain swelling, and inflammation of the pancreas and heart muscle.

In addition to pseudosugars, we now have "fake fats." Partially hydrogenated oil does not occur in nature but in the laboratory, when liquid vegetable fats are turned into solids by pumping hydrogen into them. This makes them more like animal fats in taste and feel, as well as in their harmful effects on the cardiovascular system; in fact, partially hydrogenated fats have been associated with higher cancer rates than saturated fats.

What have studies shown about artificial sweeteners?

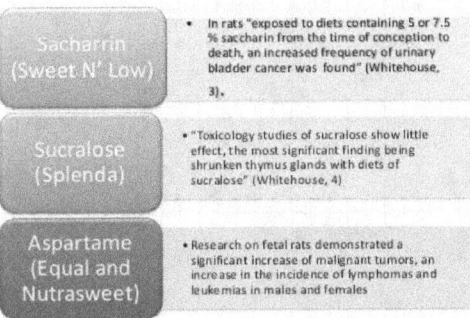

Sacharrin (Sweet N' Low)	• In rats "exposed to diets containing 5 or 7.5 % saccharin from the time of conception to death, an increased frequency of urinary bladder cancer was found" (Whitehouse, 3).
Sucralose (Splenda)	• "Toxicology studies of sucralose show little effect, the most significant finding being shrunken thymus glands with diets of sucralose" (Whitehouse, 4)
Aspartame (Equal and Nutrasweet)	• Research on fetal rats demonstrated a significant increase of malignant tumors, an increase in the incidence of lymphomas and leukemias in males and females

Trans-fatty acids (TFAs) are formed when unsaturated fatty acids (the building blocks of fat) are deformed by certain heat or chemical treatments. These deformed fats may be toxic. TFAs in the diet may damage the regulatory machinery of the body, significantly compromising health. Despite these concerns, partially hydrogenated oils and TFAs are found in a wide range of processed foods, including almost all margarines, mass-produced breads, convenience foods, and junk foods, as well as some baby foods.

For a variety of reasons, including productivity, efficiency, convenience, profit, arrogance, and curiosity, we have found abundant ways to change the nature of our diets and the nature of the animals and plants that feed us. As a group, the U.S. population eats high on the food chain, consuming unprecedented amounts of meat, chicken, fish, dairy products, fat, salt, and sugar.

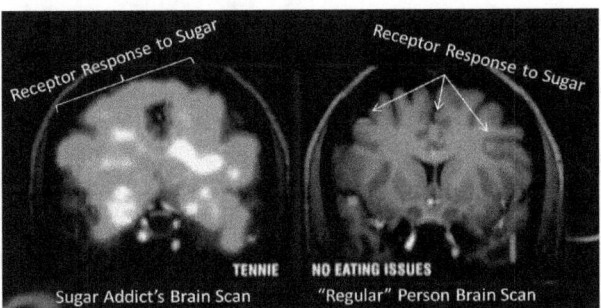

Sugar Addict's Brain Scan — TENNIE   NO EATING ISSUES — "Regular" Person Brain Scan

We cover our food with artificial chemicals while it is grown, processed, preserved, and genetically altered in ways that have only recently been introduced on this planet. After hundreds of thousands of years of evolution, during which our bodies became perfectly adapted to drawing nutrition from the natural environment, we have suddenly introduced large quantities of new, artificial substances into our diets, hoping to improve on nature.

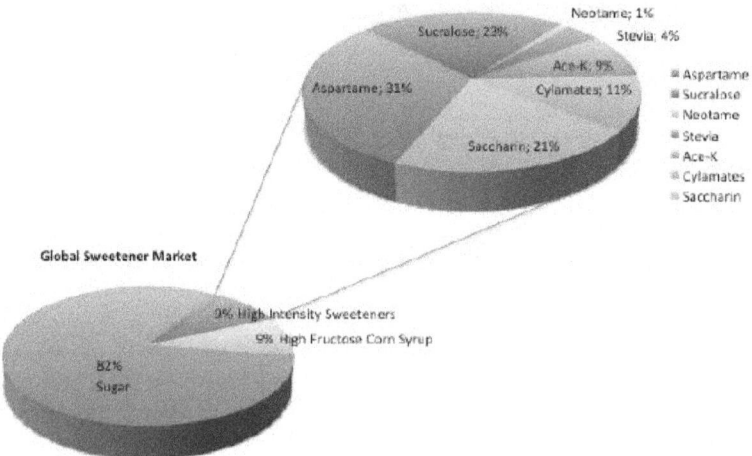

Regulation of Food Ingredients and Food Additives

Manufacturers of all foods and food additives are legally obligated to assure the public that their products are safe. For conventional foods the FFDCA requires that the food and all ingredients not be "ordinarily injurious." Ingredients with a long history of use are assumed safe, and such food items may be marketed without prior FDA approval. Cookies made with flour, brown sugar, eggs, butter, and baking soda would meet this standard.

In 1960 the FFDCA was expanded to create two legal classes of food additives as described below.

1. *Generally recognized as safe (GRAS):* The GRAS list includes all food additives and ingredients that were marketed before 1958. The GRAS list includes thousands of additives. One example is the yellow coloring added to margarine that has been in use since the 1930s. Under the law a food is unsafe if an additive "may render injurious" the food product. Food processors are not required to obtain FDA approval to use GRAS list additives; however, the presumed safety of these additives was based on their wide prior use; most were not tested. In 1977 Congress directed the FDA to begin testing the additives on the list, and this is continuing.

2. *Food additives developed since 1958:* For these additives the same legal standard of "may render injurious" applies, but they must undergo rigid testing before approval is obtained. Splenda® (sucralose), went through the FDA approval process and is now being sold.

Dietary Supplements

Dietary supplements enjoy a very favorable legal status. In 1994 Congress passed the Dietary Supplement Health and Education Act (DSHEA), which effectively deregulated the dietary supplement industry. All substances marketed as supplements prior to 1994 were assumed to be safe, whether or not research evidence existed to support this claim. The dietary supplement industry markets thousands of products containing vitamins, minerals, herbs, botanical compounds, Asian medicinal herbals, and related substances.

Under the law these supplements are classified as neither foods nor drugs. No scientific testing that demonstrates either product safety or effectiveness is required. For supplement ingredients developed after 1994, the safety standard is simply that there be no "unreasonable risk." The manufacturer must notify the FDA before marketing such a product, but no prior approval is required.

The DSHEA is a controversial law. Dietary supplements are a major industry, with large advertising budgets and a wide range of products, from single vitamins to complex mixtures. Although a dietary supplement cannot claim to cure a disease, statements about how the human body will respond to the supplement, such as a claim that it will make you burn away unwanted fat, require no substantiating evidence.

Supplements containing growth hormone or other potentially dangerous substances said to restore youthful vitality are often marketed to older adults. Steps are urgently needed to ensure consumer safety and honest claims describing appropriate use, expected effects, recommended dose, and potential interactions among drugs, herbs, and nutrients.

Agricultural Chemicals

Agricultural chemicals control destructive insects and weeds, improve seed sprouting to increase yield, prevent plant diseases, and improve market quality. However, overuse adds to food pesticide residues and farm workers' exposure to such chemicals. Researchers are helping farmers reduce their use of chemical pesticides through integrated pest management, which uses the natural enemies of insect pests to decrease their population.

The FDA has the task of assessing health risks and establishing guidelines for the thousands of agricultural chemicals in development and use.

Organic farming—which bars the use of chemical pesticides and herbicides—is growing in status as consumers become more concerned about the conditions surrounding the production of their food. Over a 10-year period, sales of organic foods grew from $3.6 billion to $21.1 billion. Organic foods are now available in most major supermarkets. Organic farmers working with soil scientists are developing sustainable systems for growing plant foods and raising beef and poultry. National standards that govern growing procedures and postharvest handling have been established for producers who wish to label their food as "organic." The USDA must certify farmers before they can use the seal of the National Organic Program

Food and Botanicals

New foods and beverages with added herbs or stimulants are blurring the distinction between food and supplements. One product receiving increased scrutiny is "energy drinks" that contain high levels of caffeine and may include added B vitamins, taurine (an amino acid), and the botanicals ginseng, gingko, or milk thistle. Energy drinks can be marketed as foods or supplements. Those sold as supplements fall under the 1994 DSHEA, enabling manufacturers to bypass label disclosure of ingredients that appear on the GRAS list, such as caffeine.

Energy drinks usually contain about 80 to 140 mg of caffeine per 8-oz serving, the equivalent of 5 oz of coffee or two cans of caffeinated soda; however, some energy drinks contain as much as 500 mg of caffeine per can—the equivalent of about 14 cans of caffeinated soda. A safe intake of caffeine is estimated to be less than 500 mg per day, although individuals with heart disease or liver disease or who take medications that slow the metabolism of caffeine need to consider a lower intake.

Energy drinks and alcohol are a particularly dangerous combination as the high caffeine content of the energy drink reduces the symptoms of intoxication, encouraging even greater alcohol consumption. Excessive energy drink consumption has been related to caffeine-induced seizures, cardiac arrhythmias, and death. Energy drinks often contain as much as 37 g of sugar per 12-oz can; young men participating in a national survey added 477 kcal per week through use of energy drinks.

The Problem of Misinformation: Food and Health

For centuries people have been concerned with the safety and wholesomeness of their food. Particular foods were 210believed to possess healing properties or, conversely, cause illness, and certain religious food laws are likely rooted in food safety. In the absence of formal health care, remedies prepared from local plants and herbs were used to cure ailments as much as possible.

In today's world of electronic communication, the Internet, blogs, and other forms of messaging can be used to advertise foods, drugs, herbs, and other plant botanicals as preventives or cures for common conditions. Some unsubstantiated beliefs about food or plant remedies or bogus drugs are harmless, but others carry serious implications for health.

False information may be embedded in folklore, built on half-truths, or stem from intentional deception.

The FDA supports a vigorous campaign to prevent and prosecute false advertising for particular foods, supplements, or medicines.

False claims usually fall within one of the following categories:

1. The food or product will cure a specific disease or condition.

2. Certain food combinations have special therapeutic effects.

3. Only "natural" foods or plant remedies can meet body needs and prevent disease.

Misleading claims about the healing properties of certain foods or other substances delay appropriate health intervention with a worsening of the illness and possible death. Patients with difficult-to-treat conditions such as cancer, diabetes, or arthritis are especially vulnerable to fraudulent claims for medicines that promise immediate cures and relief from pain.

Diagnostic tests sold online are often the products of illegal pharmaceutical operations and result in inaccurate findings that delay treatment or lead to expenditures for unneeded medications from the same online supplier. Products formulated under unsanitary conditions or that contain potentially harmful substances can lead to further illness and critical consequences.

Misleading advertising has a high economic cost. As much as $25.2 billion per year is spent on dietary supplements, and many are unnecessary or ineffective.

Government Agencies Responsible for Food Education

Just as several federal agencies share responsibility for food safety, so several groups partner to provide food and health information to the public. The U.S. Department of Health and Human Services (USDHHS) is the major source of health information. The USDA focuses on food and diet with responsibility for the *Dietary Guidelines for Americans* and MyPlate (choosemyplate.gov). The FDA oversees consumer food and drug education and reviews food labels, food health claims, and false advertising.

Food Labels

The nutrition facts label enables consumers to compare the nutritional value of one product with another and make informed choices. The information on the original nutrition facts label is described below:

Nutrition Facts	
Serving Size 1 cup (228g)	
Servings Per Container 2	Start here
Amount Per Serving	
Calories 250 Calories from Fat 110	Check calories
% Daily Value*	Quick guide to % DV
Total Fat 12g	18%	5% or less is low
Saturated Fat 3g	15%	20% or more is high
Trans Fat 3g	
Cholesterol 30mg	10%
Sodium 470mg	20%	Limit these
Potassium 700mg	20%
Total Carbohydrate 31g	10%	Get enough of these
Dietary Fiber 0g	0%
Sugars 5g	
Protein 5g	
Vitamin A	4%
Vitamin C	2%
Calcium	20%
Iron	4%	Footnote

• *Food amount and energy content:* Food amount is described by weight, serving size, and number of servings in the package or container.

• *Macronutrient content:* Protein, carbohydrate, and fat are listed in grams. Individual amounts of saturated fat, *trans* fat, and cholesterol are also required, and some processors have voluntarily added monounsaturated and polyunsaturated fats. Total carbohydrate is broken down into dietary fiber and sugar. Suggested daily intakes are compared with reference diets of 2000 or 2500 kcal.

• *Vitamin and mineral content:* Sodium and four leader nutrients—vitamin A, vitamin C, calcium, and iron—are required on the original nutrition label. Sodium is listed in milligrams and as a percentage of the suggested upper limit of 2400 mg, the recognized goal at that time. Vitamins and minerals appear as percentages of the Daily Reference Value (DV).

The DVs were derived from the1968 edition of the Recommended Dietary Allowances (RDAs), the standards in general use when the original nutrition label was being developed. The DV represented the highest RDA for that nutrient among the various age and gender groups. For example, the DV for iron is 18 mg, the RDA for women of childbearing age. Fortified foods such as cereals also list other vitamins and minerals added in the manufacturing process.

Proposed Changes in the Nutrition Facts Label

Since the original nutrition facts label was introduced in 1994, there have been changes in our knowledge of nutrition science and the food patterns and health of the American people.

The prevalence of obesity has escalated across all age groups, and foods high in energy value and added sugars but low in nutrient density constitute a growing proportion of the American diet.

Portion sizes have increased such that the reference servings used in the development of the original nutrition label no longer represent what individuals actually eat. The proposed nutrition facts label addresses these issues as described further on.

Label Changes Based on New Nutrition Science

• **Added sugars.** The 2010 Dietary Guidelines for Americans recommended that consumers limit their intakes of added sugars, and the meal plans provided on MyPlate (choosemyplate.gov) include an upper limit to intake of added sugars. The original nutrition label indicates the total amount of sugar in a food but does not indicate what portion is naturally occurring sugar and what portion is added sugars. The proposed label provides consumers with the amount of added sugar and the total sugar (naturally occurring sugar plus added sugar) in the food.

• **Fats.** The proposed food label will continue to note the amounts of total fat, saturated fat, and *trans* fats in a food, but it will not list the total calories coming from fat. Current research suggests that the type of fat in the diet is more important to health than the number of calories obtained from fat.

• **Specific nutrients.** The original nutrition label drew attention to calcium, iron, vitamin A, and vitamin C, problem nutrients at that time. Recent U.S. dietary surveys have revealed that many population groups are deficient in calcium, iron, vitamin D, and potassium, nutrients with important roles in the prevention of chronic disease, and these nutrients will be mandatory on the proposed label. Vitamin A and vitamin C intakes are generally adequate in most U.S. population groups and will no longer be mandatory, although they may be added.

• **Daily Reference Value (DV).** The DV serves two purposes: it establishes a maximum intake for a nutrient such as fat, and it indicates the percentage of the daily requirement of a nutrient, such as calcium, that is provided in a serving. The DVs for several nutrients, including sodium and calcium, are being revised to agree with current Dietary Reference Intakes (DRIs). The maximum intake for sodium will be lowered from 2400 mg to 2300 mg, and the DV for calcium will increase from 1000 mg to 1300 mg.

Label Changes Pertaining to Serving Sizes and Labeling Requirements

• *Reference servings.* The size of food portions consumed by the U.S. population has increased greatly over the past 20 years, and so have the calories and nutrients that go with them. By law reference servings used on nutrition labels must reflect what individuals actually eat, not what dietitians recommend they eat; thus 27 of the 158 reference servings used in labeling will be adjusted to accommodate current eating patterns. Several new reference servings will be developed for use with new foods.

• *Number of servings in a package.* The size and number of servings contained in a package as stated on the original nutrition label were often misunderstood. A food package perceived by the general public to contain a 1-cup single serving that was typically eaten in one sitting could be labeled as containing two, ½ cup servings; consequently the portion actually consumed contained twice the calories expected. The proposed nutrition label will require that packages containing between 150% and 200% of the reference serving, such as a 20-ounce can of soda or a 15-ounce can of soup, must be labeled as containing one serving.

Packages containing at least 200% but less than or equal to 400% of the reference serving will require dual labeling, listing information per serving and per package

Food, Glucose and the Body

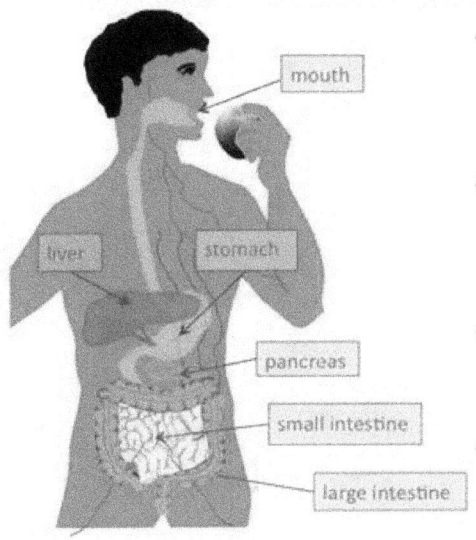

- Glucose comes from food that contains carbohydrate (eg, starch, sugar, rice, pasta, bread, cakes, etc.)

- The mouth, the stomach and the small intestine digest (break down) food to glucose

- Glucose enters the blood stream from the small intestine

- The blood then carries glucose to muscles and the brain

*****

Chapter Seven.... Nutritional and Energy Health!

*****

The Nutritional Health of an individual is known as his or her *Nutritional Status* and describes how well their specific Nutrient needs are being met. Nutritional Status is influenced by living situation, social and economic factors, available food, food choices, and state of health.

Nutritional status differs from *dietary status.*

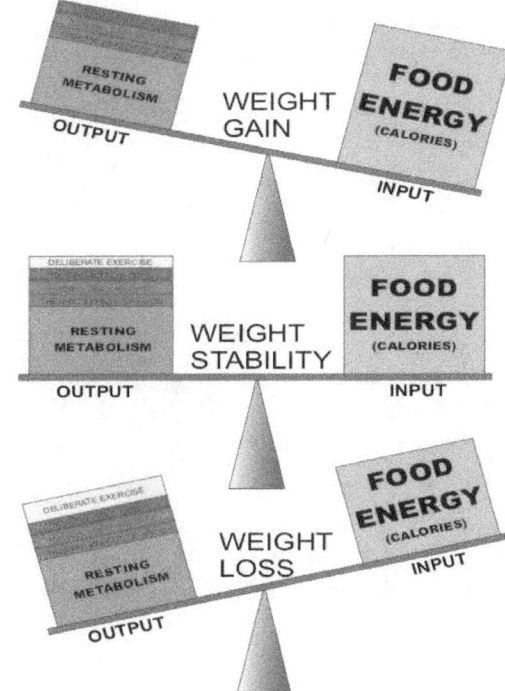

Evaluating Nutritional Status requires a combination of Dietary, Biochemical, **Anthropometric**, and clinical measurements, whereas Dietary Status focuses only on what foods are being consumed and their Nutrient content.

It is important to know not only what an individual is eating, but also whether the Body is Absorbing and making use of those Nutrients. This helps us distinguish between a *Primary Nutrient Deficiency* and a *Secondary Nutrient Deficiency.*

A Primary Nutrient Deficiency is caused by insufficient dietary intake of a particular Nutrient or combination of Nutrients.

A Secondary Nutrient Deficiency is the result of poor absorption or metabolism of a specific Nutrient caused by an interfering substance, a disease or condition, or an elevated requirement.

Blood Nutrient levels can help identify a Nutrient deficiency or a Nutrient excess brought about by overuse of highly fortified foods or dietary supplements, although this is not true for all Nutrients.

Body weight for height and other anthropometric measurements provide estimates of the proportion of body fat versus lean body mass.

An evaluation of nutritional status usually includes related conditions associated with food and nutrient intake, such as diabetes and obesity, or osteoporosis and calcium

Nutrient Density

A major factor in Nutritional Health is the *Nutrient Density* of our diet.

This term refers to the relative quality and value of the Nutrient Content of a food in relation to the quality and value of its Energy Content.

A **Nutrient Dense** food contributes Vitamins, Minerals, Essential Fatty Acids, and/or Protein to the diet in addition to KCalories (Energy).

Energy Content is the amount of KCalories available for Energy production.

A food that is not Nutrient Dense adds KCalories but lacks other Nutrients.

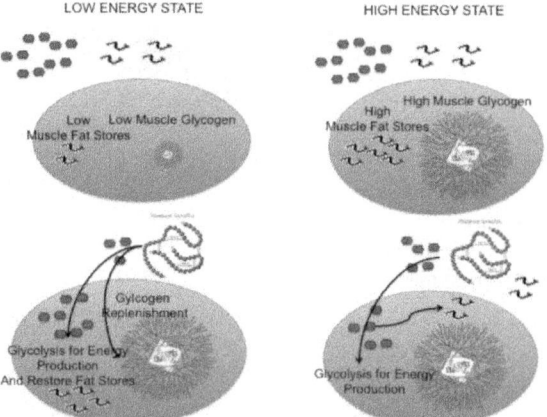

LOW ENERGY STATE   HIGH ENERGY STATE

Insulin in a "low energy" state drives glucose and FA uptake while shifting metabolism to carbohydrate

In a "high energy" state, Insulin signals carbohydrate Metabolism and fatty acid synthesis

As an example, we take a look at 3 types of foods. The first is a hamburger, which is made from lean ground beef supplies protein and although it adds some Fat which can be utilized as Energy, it presents NO Life Energy.

Fruits and vegetables are high in Vitamins and Minerals and low in KCalories and are Nutrient dense.

In contrast, a doughnut is high in KCalories and adds primarily Sugar and Fat, and sugar-sweetened soft drinks add only kcalories. These food-like items are considered to be **"empty calories"** as they contribute no Essential Nutrients or Life Energy.

Many Americans who are overweight or obese exhibit undernutrition because the foods they consume are not Nutrient Dense and manifest little to no Life Energy.

Malnutrition

Malnutrition or ***Malnourishment*** is a condition that results from eating a diet in which nutrients are either not enough or are too much such that the diet causes health problems. It may involve Calories, Protein, Carbohydrates, Vitamins or Minerals. Not enough Nutrients is referred to as Undernutrition or Undernourishment, while too much is called Over-nutrition.

Malnutrition is often used specifically to refer to undernutrition where there is not enough Calories, Protein, or Micronutrients. If undernutrition occurs during pregnancy, or before two years of age, it may result in permanent problems with physical and mental development. Extreme Undernourishment, known as starvation, may have symptoms that include: a short height, thin body, very poor energy levels, and swollen legs and abdomen. People also often get infections and are frequently cold. The symptoms of Micronutrient Deficiencies depend on the micronutrient that is lacking.

There were 793 million Undernourished people in the world in 2015 (13% of the total population). This is a reduction of 216 million people since 1990 when 23% were Undernourished. In 2012 it was estimated that another billion people had a lack of Vitamins and Minerals. In 2013, Protein-Energy Malnutrition was estimated to have resulted in 469,000 deaths—down from 510,000 deaths in 1990. Other Nutritional deficiencies, which include Iodine deficiency and Iron deficiency Anemia, result in another 84,000 deaths.

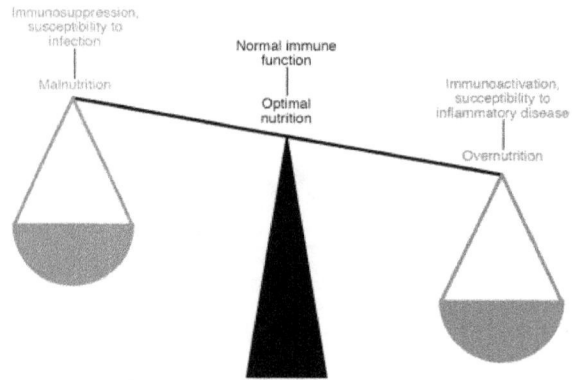

In 2010, malnutrition was the cause of 1.4% of all disability adjusted life years. About a third of deaths in children are believed to be due to Undernutrition, although the deaths are rarely labelled as such. In 2010, it was estimated to have contributed to about 1.5 million deaths in women and children, though some estimate the number may be greater than 3 million. An additional 165 million children were estimated to have stunted growth from malnutrition in 2013

Undernutrition: Undernutrition subsequent to insufficient intake; altered digestion; or absorption of protein, energy, or both (calories); is called *Protein-Energy Malnutrition (PEM)* or *Protein-Calorie Malnutrition (PCM)*. Characteristics include weight loss, fat loss, muscle wasting and weakness, impaired immune function, poor wound healing, and reduction of protein synthesis.

Undernutrition takes various forms ranging from marginal nutritional status to the emaciated famine victim. Persons with *Marginal Nutritional Status* are meeting their minimum day-to-day nutritional needs but lack the nutrient stores to cope with any added physiologic or metabolic demand arising from injury or illness, pregnancy, or growth spurt. Marginal Nutritional Status results from poor eating habits, stressful environments, or insufficient resources to obtain appropriate types or amounts of food.

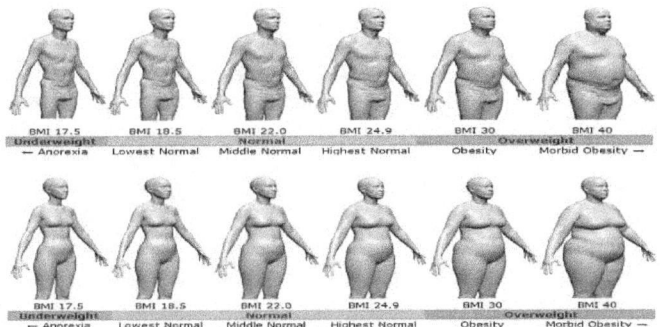

Current U.S. food trends add to the risk of marginal nutritional status or undernutrition among all age groups. Money spent for food away from home has increased, while money spent for food eaten at home has decreased by almost half. Meals away from home, especially those obtained at fast-food restaurants, tend to be high in TOXIC Fat, Sodium, and added Sugar, but severely nutritionally limited in Calcium, Fiber, Whole Grains, Fruits, and green, yellow, and orange vegetables.

Foods contributing the most KCalories to the diets of persons ages 2 and over are grain-based desserts (cookies, cake, doughnuts, and granola bars), followed by yeast breads, chicken and chicken-mixed dishes, sugar-sweetened soft drinks, and pizza. Sugar-sweetened soft drinks and fruit drinks supply almost half of the added sugar in the U.S. diet, and sugar intakes are 10 times higher than recommended in the 2010 *Dietary Guidelines for Americans.*

Added sugar contributes 316 KCal per day to the average diet and is believed by some Nutrition experts to be a major contributor to the Obesity epidemic and rise in type 2 Diabetes. Despite an abundance of KCalories, most Americans are deficient in Calcium, Vitamin D, Fiber, and Potassium.

$$\text{BMI} = \text{Weight in kilograms} / (\text{Height in meters})^2$$
or
$$\text{BMI} = \left[\text{Weight in pounds} / (\text{Height in inches})^2\right] \times 703$$

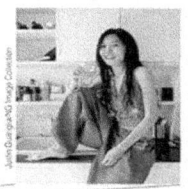

Being underweight is associated with increased risk of early death, but this does not mean that all thin people are at risk.[1] People who are naturally lean have a lower incidence of certain chronic diseases and do not face increased health risks due to their low body weight. However, low body fat due to starvation, eating disorders, or a disease process decreases energy reserves and the ability of the immune system to fight disease.

To find your BMI, locate your height in the leftmost column and read across to your weight. Follow the column containing your weight up to the top line to find your BMI. A BMI < 18.5 kg/m² is classified as **underweight**, a BMI ≥ 25 and < 30 kg/m² is classified as overweight, and a BMI ≥ 30 kg/m² is classified as obese. A BMI ≥ 40 kg/m² is considered **extreme obesity or morbid obesity**.[1]

Height	UNDER-WEIGHT		NORMAL						OVERWEIGHT					OBESE										EXTREME OBESITY		
BMI	17	18	19	20	21	22	23	24	25	26	27	28	29	30	31	32	33	34	35	36	37	38	39	40	41	42
4'10"	81	86	91	96	100	105	110	115	119	124	129	134	138	143	148	153	158	162	167	172	177	181	186	191	196	201
4'11"	84	89	94	99	104	109	114	119	124	128	133	138	143	148	153	158	163	168	173	178	183	188	193	198	203	208
5'0"	87	92	97	102	107	112	118	123	128	133	138	143	148	153	158	163	168	174	179	184	189	194	199	204	209	215
5'1"	90	95	100	106	111	116	122	127	132	137	143	148	153	158	164	169	174	180	185	190	195	201	206	211	217	222
5'2"	93	98	104	109	115	120	126	131	136	142	147	153	158	164	169	175	180	186	191	196	202	207	213	218	224	229
5'3"	96	102	107	113	118	124	130	135	141	146	152	158	163	169	175	180	186	191	197	203	208	214	220	225	231	237
5'4"	99	105	110	116	122	128	134	140	145	151	157	163	169	174	180	186	192	197	204	209	215	221	227	232	238	244
5'5"	102	108	114	120	126	132	138	144	150	156	162	168	174	180	186	192	198	204	210	216	222	228	234	240	246	252
5'6"	105	112	118	124	130	136	142	148	155	161	167	173	179	186	192	198	204	210	216	223	229	235	241	247	253	260
5'7"	108	115	121	127	134	140	146	153	159	166	172	178	185	191	198	204	211	217	223	230	236	242	249	255	261	268
5'8"	112	119	125	131	138	144	151	158	164	171	177	184	190	197	203	210	216	223	230	236	243	249	256	262	269	276
5'9"	115	122	128	135	142	149	155	162	169	176	182	189	196	203	209	216	223	230	236	243	250	257	263	270	277	284
5'10"	119	126	132	139	146	153	160	167	174	181	188	195	202	209	216	222	229	236	243	250	257	264	271	278	285	292
5'11"	122	129	136	143	150	157	165	172	179	186	193	200	208	215	222	229	236	243	250	257	265	272	279	286	293	301
6'0"	125	133	140	147	154	162	169	177	184	191	199	206	213	221	228	235	242	250	258	265	272	279	287	294	302	309
6'1"	129	137	144	151	159	166	174	182	189	197	204	212	219	227	235	242	250	257	265	272	280	288	295	302	310	318
6'2"	132	140	148	155	163	171	179	186	194	202	210	218	225	233	241	249	256	264	272	280	287	295	303	311	319	326
6'3"	135	144	152	160	168	176	184	192	200	208	216	224	232	240	248	256	264	272	279	287	295	303	311	319	327	335
6'4"	140	148	156	164	172	180	189	197	205	213	221	230	238	246	254	263	271	279	287	295	304	312	320	328	336	344

Someone who is overweight based on BMI but consumes a healthy diet and exercises regularly may be more fit and at lower risk for chronic diseases than someone with a BMI in the healthy range who is sedentary and eats a poor diet.

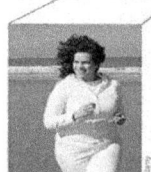
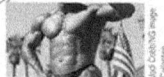
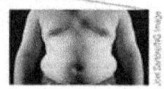

A high BMI may be caused by either too much body fat or a large amount of muscle. Therefore, in muscular athletes, BMI does not provide an accurate estimate of health risk. Both of these individuals have a BMI of 33, but only the man on the right has excess body fat. The high body weight of the man on the left is due to his large muscle mass. His body fat, and hence his risk of obesity-related health problems, is low.

Public health nutritionists describe the American diet as energy rich but nutrient poor. Although persons with less-than-optimal intakes of micronutrients may not suffer from overt malnutrition, they are at greater risk of physical illness than those who are well nourished. The body can adapt to marginal nutrient intake but any added physiologic stress that calls on nutrient stores will result in overt malnutrition.

Over-nutrition: More than two thirds of American adults are overweight or obese, making these conditions the two most common forms of Over-nutrition.

Overweight is defined as body mass index (BMI) greater than **25** and obesity as BMI greater than **30**. Both are associated with a number of health risks including coronary heart disease, type 2 diabetes mellitus, certain cancers (breast, endometrial, colon), hypertension, dyslipidemia, stroke, gallbladder disease, liver disease, sleep apnea, osteoarthritis, and infertility.

Over-nutrition takes various forms. Excessive energy intake coupled with low physical activity leads to unwanted weight gain and elevated health risks for conditions such as metabolic syndrome. Over-nutrition also occurs with excessive intakes of Micronutrients from overuse of dietary supplements. Inappropriate amounts of particular Vitamins or Minerals damage tissues and interfere with the absorption and metabolism of other essential nutrients. Herbal preparations, growing in popularity, carry the potential for harmful interactions with nutrients or medications

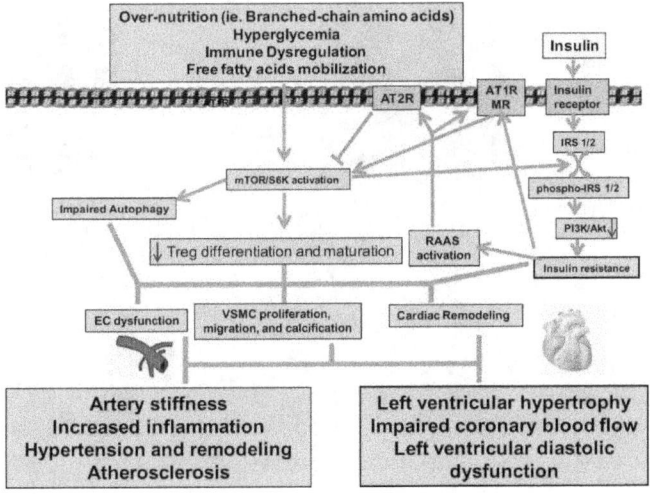

What Is Body Composition?

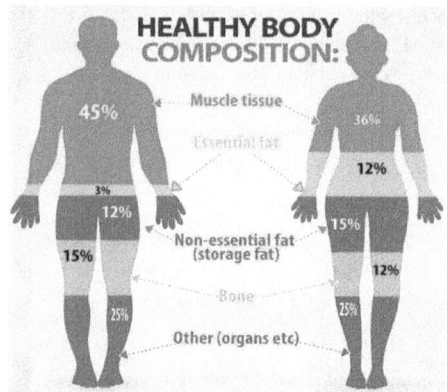

Nothing is or can be more personal than our own Body. And nothing has a greater influence over how long that Body functions properly than its composition. **Body composition** is the ratio of Muscle Mass in relations to Fat Mass.

Body composition is the term used to describe the different components that, when taken together, make up a person's body weight.

Our Human body is composed of a variety of different tissue types including Lean Tissues (Muscle, Bone, and other Organs) that are Metabolically Active, and Fat (Adipose) Tissue that is not.

Muscle Mass is composed of muscle, bone, organs, and other tissues of the body.

Fat Mass is the total amount of essential and storage fat in the body.

The ideal weight and Fat-Lean ratio varies considerably for men and women and by age, but the minimum percent of body fat considered safe for good health is 5 percent for Males and 12% for Females.

The average adult body fat is closer to 15 to 18% for men and 22 to 25% for women.

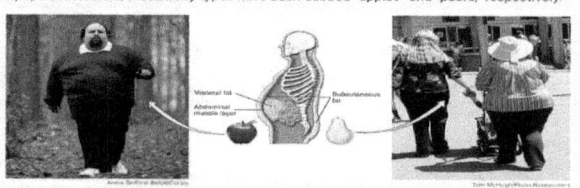

People who carry their excess fat around and above the waist have more visceral fat. Those who carry their extra fat below the waist, in the hips and thighs, have more subcutaneous fat. In the popular literature, these body types have been dubbed "apples" and "pears," respectively.

Waist circumference is indicative of the amount of visceral fat, the type of fat that is associated with increased health risk. Waist measurements along with BMI are used to estimate the health risk associated with excess body fat. These waist circumference "cutpoints" are not useful in patients with a BMI of 35 kg/m² or greater.

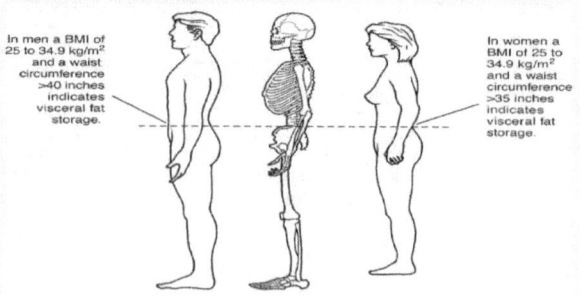

In men a BMI of 25 to 34.9 kg/m² and a waist circumference >40 inches indicates visceral fat storage.

In women a BMI of 25 to 34.9 kg/m² and a waist circumference >35 inches indicates visceral fat storage.

Essential Body Fat

Your <u>**Essential Body Fat**</u> resides in your Nerve Cells, Muscles, and Bone Marrow, as well as in your Lungs, Heart, Liver, and Intestines. It has many important functions:

- Keeps your physiological activity normal (e.g., nerve conduction)

- Helps keep your body warm

- Protects your organs from injury

- Stores energy needed when your body is active or when you are injured or ill

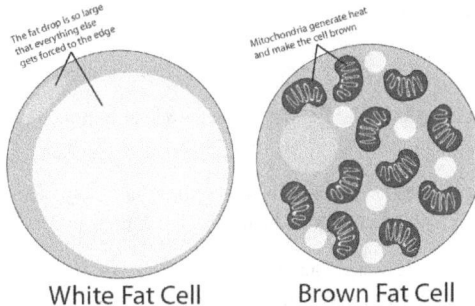

White Fat Cell   Brown Fat Cell

The desirable amount of essential fat for a healthy person is:

- Adult women: 8% to 12% of total body weight

- Adult men: 3% to 5% of total body weight

   Women have more essential body Fat in their Hips, Thighs, Breasts, and Uterus.

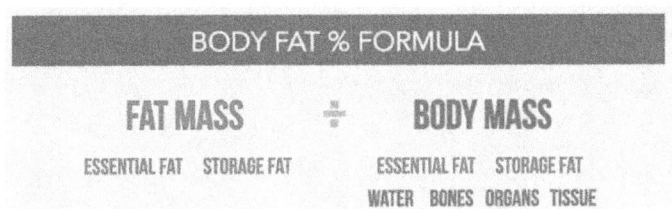

BODY FAT % FORMULA

FAT MASS ÷ **BODY MASS**

ESSENTIAL FAT STORAGE FAT   ESSENTIAL FAT STORAGE FAT
                                 WATER BONES ORGANS TISSUE

Storage Fat

Storage Fat is essentially Potential Energy. Some Fat besides what is considered Essential is also desirable on our Bodies. In addition to offering Organ Protection and Body Insulation, this **Storage Fat** supplies what can be considered as Emergency Energy: 3500 KCalories per pound of Adipose Tissue.

General Body Fat Percentage Categories		
Classification:	**Women:**	**Men:**
Essential Fat	10 - 12%	2 - 4%
Athletes	14 - 20%	6 - 13%
Fitness	21 - 24%	14 - 17%
Acceptable	25 - 31%	18 - 25%
At Risk	32% plus	25% plus

For these purposes, Storage Fat is termed 'Emergency' because our Bodies wouldn't have a chance to 'Burn' the Adipose Tissue to release the Energy unless we stopped eating – as in a FAST.

BALANCE is the Key. Too little and we will lack this vital Energy source; Too much and we get weighed-down right to the grave.

There are a variety of methods that exist for determining whether body composition places a person at risk for disease.

Some methods are simple calculations and are based on the relationship between the person's height and weight. Other methods look specifically at the fat contained in the body.

Obesity is not just an American problem but also a growing concern worldwide. It is such an important trend that the term *Globesity* has been coined to reflect the escalation of global obesity and overweight.

Around the world, approximately 1.4 billion adults are overweight, and of these, 500 million are obese; more than 10% of the world's adult population. Once considered a problem only in high-income countries, overweight and obesity are now on the rise in low- and middle-income countries, particularly in urban settings.

What's Wrong with Having Too Much Body Fat?

Having too much body fat increases the risk of developing a host of chronic health problems, including high blood pressure, heart disease, high blood cholesterol, diabetes, gallbladder disease, liver disease, arthritis, sleep disorders, respiratory problems, menstrual irregularities, and cancers of the breast, uterus, prostate, and colon.

Obesity also increases the incidence and severity of infectious disease and has been linked to poor wound healing and surgical complications.

The more excess body fat you have, the greater your health risks.

The longer you carry excess fat, the greater the risks; individuals who gain excess weight at a young age and remain overweight throughout life face the greatest health risks.

Chest Fat: High Estrogen, Low Testosterone

Belly Fat: High Insulin/Low Growth Hormone/Low or High Estrogen/High testosterone/High Cortisol

Love Handle Fat: High Insulin and Blood Sugar Imbalance

Hips, Butt and Thigh Fat: High Estrogen, Low Progesterone, Low Growth Hormone

Arm Fat: High Insulin, Low DHEA

Chest Fat: High Estrogen, Low Testosterone

Arm Fat: High Insulin, Low DHEA

Abdominal Fat: High Insulin/Low Growth Hormone/ High Estrogen/Low Testosterone/High Cortisol

Love Handle Fat: High Insulin and Blood Sugar Imbalance

Hips, Butt and Thigh Fat: High Estrogen, Low Growth Hormone

What is the Best Prediction Equation to Determine Energy Needs?

Assessment of energy needs is a necessary component in the Nutrition Care Process (NCP). Indirect calorimetry is the "gold standard" for determining resting metabolic rate (RMR) and is accurate within 5% in most cases. However, because indirect calorimetry is not always available, prediction equations are commonly used to determine RMR.

The four prediction equations most commonly used in clinical practice are as follows:

Mifflin-St. Jeor	
Men	RMR = (9.99 × wt in kg) + (6.25 × ht in cm) − (4.92 × age in yr) + 5
Women	RMR = (9.99 × wt in kg) + (6.25 × ht in cm) − (4.92 × age in yr) − 161

Harris-Benedict	
Men	RMR = 66.47 + (13.75 × wt in kg) + (5.0 × ht in cm) − (6.75 × age in yr)
Women	RMR = 665.09 + (9.56 × wt in kg) + (1.84 × ht in cm) − (4.67 × age in yr)

Owen	
Men	RMR = 879 + (10.2 × wt in kg)
Women	RMR = 795 + (7.18 × wt in kg)

World Health Organization/Food & Agriculture Organization/United Nations University (WHO/FAO/UNU)	
Weight Only (Age [yr])	
Men	
18-30	15.3 × wt in kg + 679
31-60	11.6 × wt in kg + 879
>60	13.5 × wt in kg + 487
Women	
18-30	14.7 × wt in kg + 496
31-60	8.7 × wt in kg + 829
>60	10.5 × wt in kg + 596
Weight & Height (m) (Age [yr])	
Men	
18-30	(15.4 × wt in kg) − (27 × ht in m) + 717
31-60	(11.3 × wt in kg) + (16 × ht in m) + 901
>60	(8.8 × wt in kg) + (1128 × ht in m) − 1071
Women	
18-30	(13.3 × wt in kg) + (34 × ht in m) + 35
31-60	(8.7 × wt in kg) − (25 × ht in m) + 865
>60	(9.2 × wt in kg) + (637 × ht in m) − 302

Of the four equations listed previously, the Mifflin-St. Jeor equation was found to be the most accurate in estimating basal metabolic rate (BMR). The oldest prediction equation in clinical use, Harris-Benedict, was found to systematically overestimate basal energy expenditure (BEE) by at least 5%. The Owen equation underestimates RMR about 21% of the time and overestimates RMR 6% of the time. Accuracy of the WHO/FAO/UNU equations could not be evaluated because of how the equations have been validated. For more details about the research of these prediction equations, please refer to the Frankenfield manuscripts cited in the bibliography.

Forms of Energy

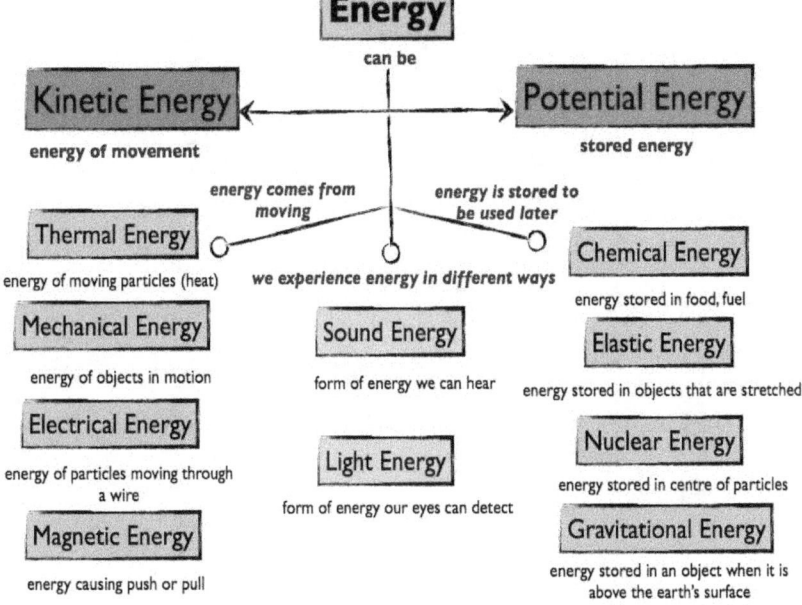

Energy

can be

Kinetic Energy ←———————→ **Potential Energy**

energy of movement   stored energy

energy comes from   energy is stored to
moving   be used later

Thermal Energy ○   **Chemical Energy**

energy of moving particles (heat)   *we experience energy in different ways*   energy stored in food, fuel

Mechanical Energy   **Sound Energy**   **Elastic Energy**

energy of objects in motion   form of energy we can hear   energy stored in objects that are stretched

Electrical Energy   **Nuclear Energy**

energy of particles moving through   **Light Energy**   energy stored in centre of particles
a wire

form of energy our eyes can detect

Magnetic Energy   **Gravitational Energy**

energy causing push or pull   energy stored in an object when it is
above the earth's surface

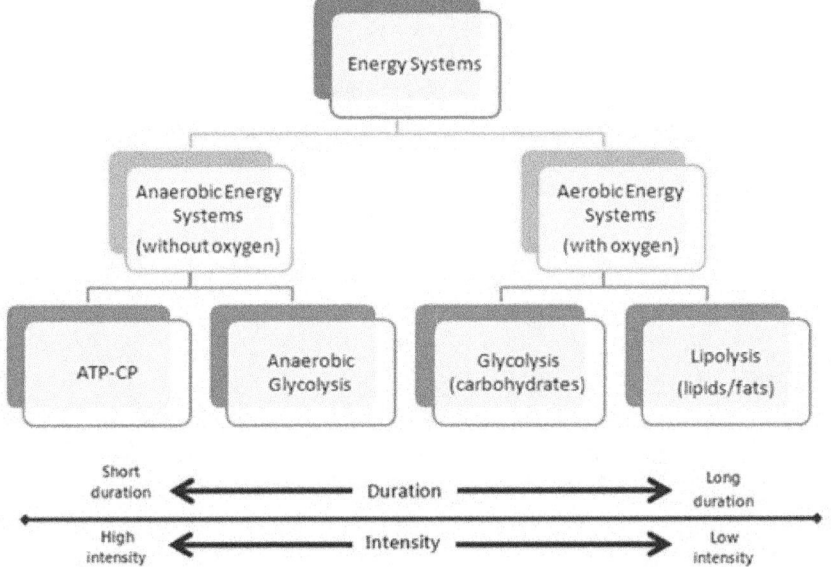

*****

Chapter Eight .... The Human Energy System!

*****

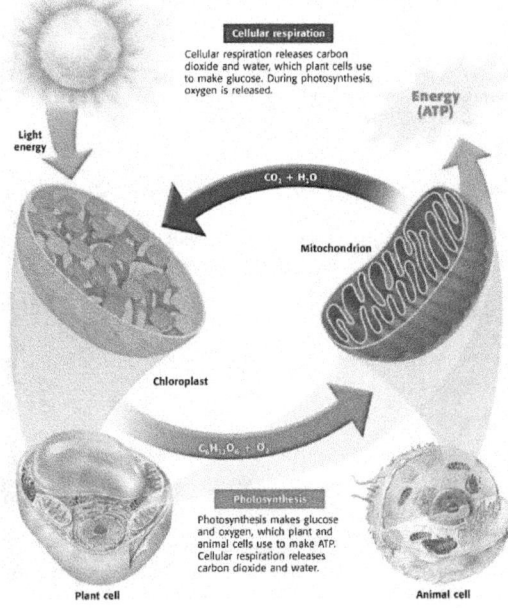

Cellular respiration

Cellular respiration releases carbon dioxide and water, which plant cells use to make glucose. During photosynthesis, oxygen is released.

Light energy

Energy (ATP)

$CO_2 + H_2O$

Mitochondrion

Chloroplast

$C_6H_{12}O_6 + O_2$

Photosynthesis

Photosynthesis makes glucose and oxygen, which plant and animal cells use to make ATP. Cellular respiration releases carbon dioxide and water.

Plant cell   Animal cell

In our Physical world, **Energy** as we discussed, like Matter, is neither Created nor Destroyed.

So when we speak of Energy being Produced, what is really meant is that Energy is being *Transformed.*

Energy constantly changes form as it moves through various systems.

In our Human body, Metabolic Reactions convert the Stored Chemical Energy in food to other forms of Energy that carry out body work.

The ultimate source of LIFE Energy is our Sun, with its vast reservoir of Heat and Light Energies.

By the process of photosynthesis Plants use Water and Carbon Dioxide (CO_2) to transform the Life Energy manifested from the Sun into Carbohydrate, a storage form of Chemical Energy of Life Energy that we can Eat. In our Bodies, these Carbohydrates are converted to Glucose, and in conjunction with Fatty Acids are Metabolized to release Energy and support our Life.

The end products of our Body Energy Metabolism is Water and CO_2.

These end products then become available to plants to produce more Carbohydrate for our use. Completing the Cycle of Life where Plants give us what we Need and We give the Plants what they need.

The Cycle Of LIFE !!!

ANIMAL MEATS ARE NOT IN OUR NUTRITIONAL OR LIFE ENERGY CYCLE !!!

Regardless to the hoopla made about Vitamin B12 only being a by-product of animal meats is TRUE......the dispute comes in with the theory that we NEED Vitamin B12 (or any other Nutrient) from consuming animal flesh.

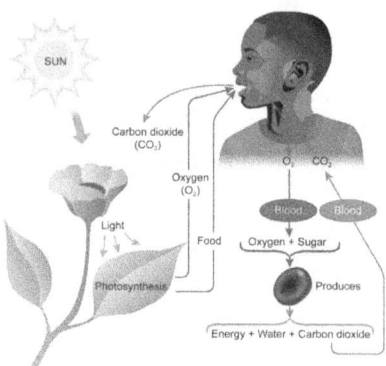

THE CONSUMPTION AND ATTEMPTED DIGESTION OF ANIMAL MEATS IS ANTI-LIFE !!!

If we never consume animal meats it doesn't prevent the Metabolism of the Life Energy in the form of Glucose. IN FACT, consuming animal meats with any Carbohydrate PROHIBITS Digestion of BOTH.

Digestion is the act of breaking the Atomic Bonds of food to release Energy and Nutrients in the form of Macro/Micro-Nutrients and KCalories.

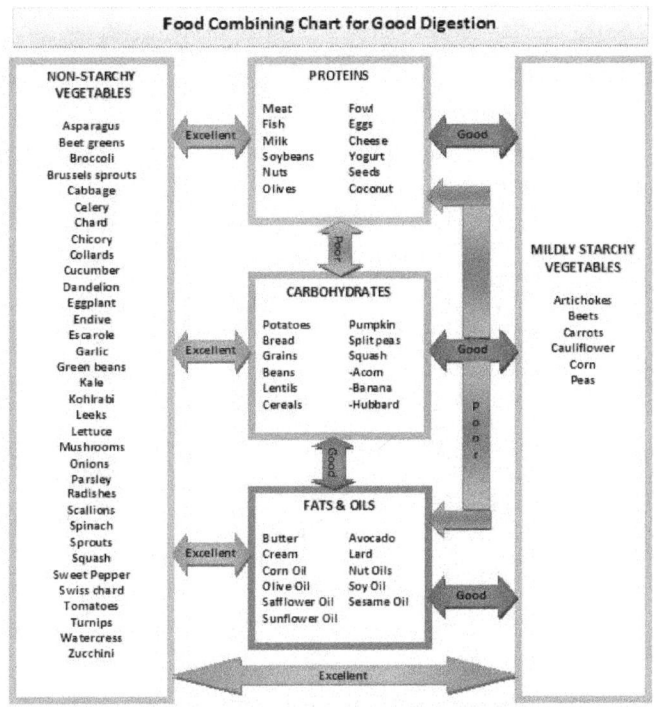

Food Combining Chart for Good Digestion

NON-STARCHY VEGETABLES

Asparagus
Beet greens
Broccoli
Brussels sprouts
Cabbage
Celery
Chard
Chicory
Collards
Cucumber
Dandelion
Eggplant
Endive
Escarole
Garlic
Green beans
Kale
Kohlrabi
Leeks
Lettuce
Mushrooms
Onions
Parsley
Radishes
Scallions
Spinach
Sprouts
Squash
Sweet Pepper
Swiss chard
Tomatoes
Turnips
Watercress
Zucchini

PROTEINS

Meat	Fowl
Fish	Eggs
Milk	Cheese
Soybeans	Yogurt
Nuts	Seeds
Olives	Coconut

CARBOHYDRATES

Potatoes	Pumpkin
Bread	Split peas
Grains	Squash
Beans	-Acorn
Lentils	-Banana
Cereals	-Hubbard

FATS & OILS

Butter	Avocado
Cream	Lard
Corn Oil	Nut Oils
Olive Oil	Soy Oil
Safflower Oil	Sesame Oil
Sunflower Oil	

MILDLY STARCHY VEGETABLES

Artichokes
Beets
Carrots
Cauliflower
Corn
Peas

Excellent · Good · Poor

Fruits are best when eaten separate from other foods on an empty stomach. It is best to eat melons and sweet fruits separately. Fruit makes an awesome breakfast and an energetic start to the day.

ACID FRUITS		SUB ACID FRUITS		SWEET FRUITS		MELONS
Lemon	Lime	Apples	Pears	Bananas	Raisins	Cantaloupe
Orange	Tangerines	Cherries	Nectarines	Grapes	Prunes	Honey dew
Raspberries	Pomegranate	Tart Grapes	Mangoes	Dried fruits	Figs	Watermelon
Pineapple	Grapefruit	Huckleberries	Sweet Plums	Dates		Casaba
Blackberries	Strawberries	Kiwi	Apricots			Musk
Kumquat	Sour Plums	Papaya	Fresh Figs			Persian
Sour apples		Peach				Crenshaw

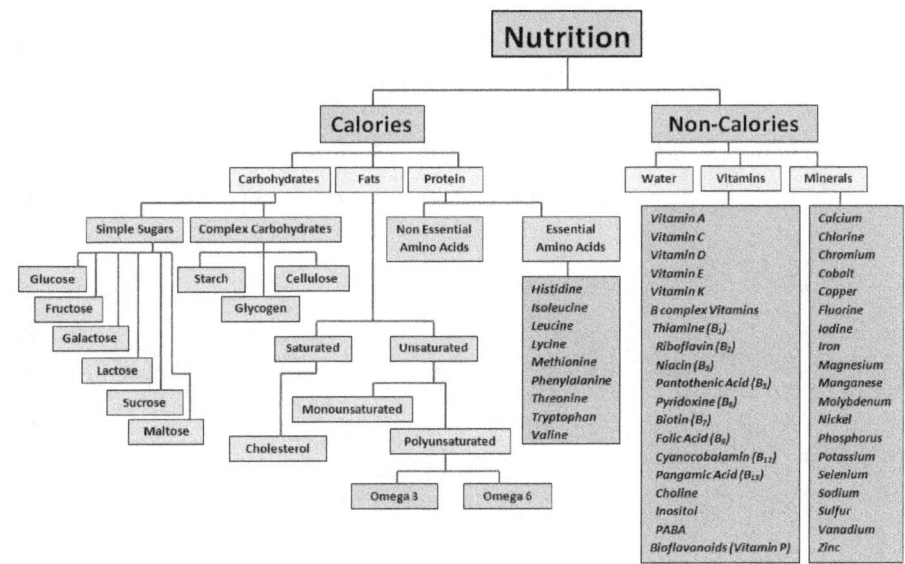

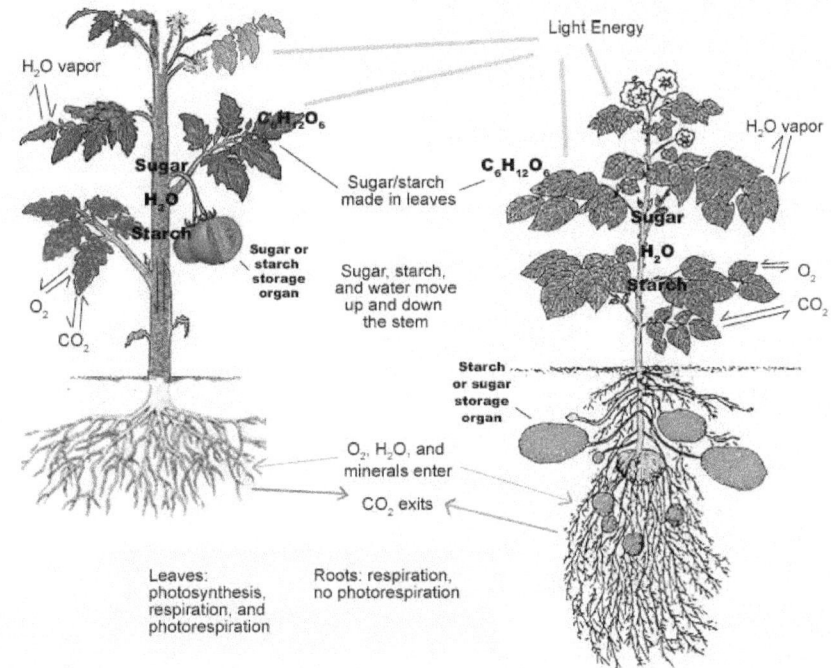

H$_2$O vapor

Light Energy

H$_2$O vapor

C$_6$H$_{12}$O$_6$

Sugar

H$_2$O

Starch

Sugar/starch
made in leaves

C$_6$H$_{12}$O$_6$

Sugar

H$_2$O

Starch

O$_2$

CO$_2$

Sugar or
starch
storage
organ

Sugar, starch,
and water move
up and down
the stem

O$_2$

CO$_2$

Starch
or sugar
storage
organ

O$_2$, H$_2$O, and
minerals enter

CO$_2$ exits

Leaves:
photosynthesis,
respiration, and
photorespiration

Roots: respiration,
no photorespiration

*****

Chapter Nine .... Transformation of Energy

*****

The LIFE Energy of the Sun is manifested in the Chemical composition of the Fruits and Veggies – which are also considered the Primary Producers in our Energy-Eco System.

It is the primary producers, which synthesize and produce the energy for the entire ecosystem. These organisms produce oxygen, too.

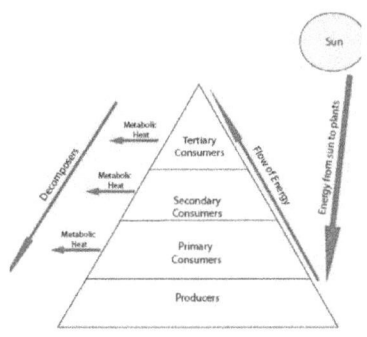

Primary producers get energy from nonliving sources. This energy is then maintained within the earth's atmosphere by organisms that eat the primary producers that hold this energy.

There are many types of primary producers within the earth's ecosystem. Plants such as trees and algae use energy from the sun and dispense it into the air and to other organisms.

Kelp, which is brown algae, and coral are two dominant primary producers. Others include protists, such as the asexual Euglena micro-organism, and phytoplankton, a main primary producer in the ocean food web. Some forms of bacteria at the sea floor's hot springs and cold vents possess the ability to produce energy through the use of inorganic molecules.

Photosynthesis

Photosynthesis is one way primary producers capture and disperse energy. The primary producers performing this task are plants, coral, bacteria and algae. Photosynthetic bacteria, such as those existing in soil cultures, are a relatively new discovery.

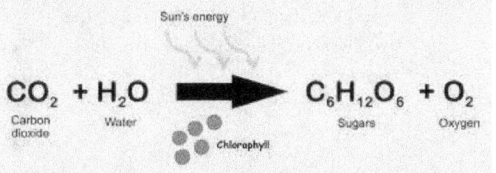

$$CO_2 + H_2O \rightarrow C_6H_{12}O_6 + O_2$$

Carbon dioxide · Water · Sugars · Oxygen · Chlorophyll

Earth's Energy Cycle. As Life Energy manifests from the Sun, the Producers, Plants, absorb this Un-Seen Energy and converts it into usable Energy.

Primary Consumers, Herbivores, then eat the Plants that contain this Life Energy. Carnivores then eat the Herbivores to obtain the limited Life Energy in them, and other animals, such as vultures, eat the feces and dead animal bodies.

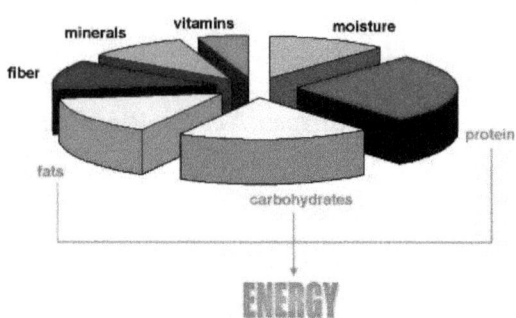

Thus, the Primary Producers begin the Energy Cycle here on our Earth. The best Quality and Value of Energy is made manifest in the form of Carbohydrates and GLUCOSE is our Life Energy provided by the Primary Producers.

For us, these forms of Energy manifests as Carbohydrates, Lipids/Fats or Protein – our MACRO-Nutrients.

Vitamins and Minerals are our MICRO-Nutrients. They are also considered Essential elements, as well as to help facilitate the Metabolizing of our Energy-yielding Macro-Nutrients, but NO Energy is manifested from them.

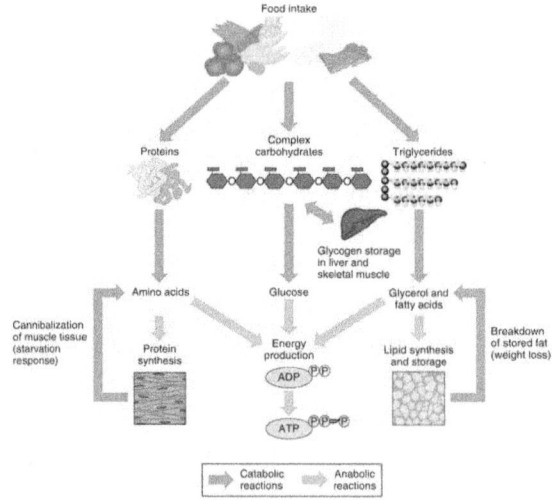

Carbohydrates, most important class of modular Molecules found in all living things, are made up of Carbon, Hydrogen, and Oxygen Atoms.

Carbohydrates play a central role in the way that living things acquire and use our Energy, and they form many of the solid structures of living things.

We use Carbohydrates literally every day in many of the foods products, the fuels we burn, the clothes you wear, and even the paper of this book.

The simplest Carbs manifest in Sugars, which are Molecules that are determined by the number of Carbon Atoms, which can be between Five, Six, or Seven Atoms, arranged in a ring-like structure. Glucose, an important Sugar in the Energy cycle of almost all Life forms. Glucose figures prominently in the Energy Metabolism of every living Cell; and it supplies the Life Energy that we use to move and grow.

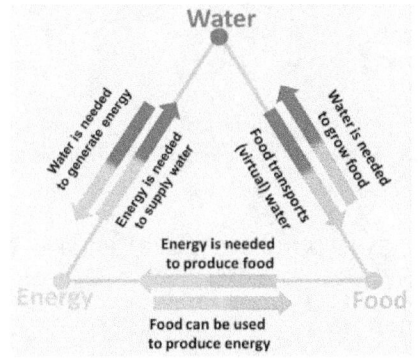

The general chemical formula for Sugar is *CnH2nOn* or *Cn(H2O)n*. Glucose, for example, has the formula **C6H12O6**. As often happens with organic molecules, other forms of the molecule have the same chemical composition but have the components arranged differently.

As an example, we show the sugar fructose, a sugar commonly found in fruit. It has the same number of carbon, hydrogen, and oxygen atoms as glu cose, but the atoms are arranged slightly differently, and this different arrangement gives fructose a different chemical behavior.

Chemists refer to individual Sugar Molecules as Monosaccharides, which means "*one sugar.*"

The Carbohydrates that we eat, however, are usually formed from only two or more Sugar Molecules. Ordinary table sugar, for example, is made from two sugars, glucose and fructose, linked together by man-made, grafted Covalent bond, which when digested releases TOXIC Energy. The opposite of the Life Energy manifested from naturally occurring Glucose.

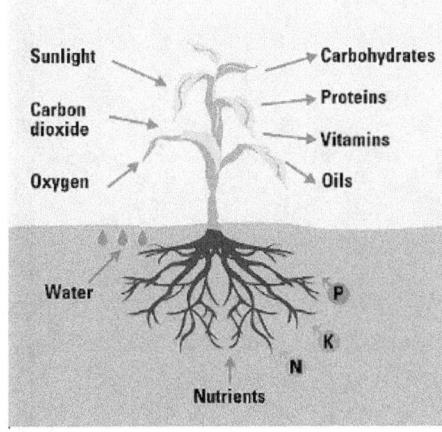

The Fruits and Veggies are created to perfectly transform and provide the necessary Life Energy for us to Grow and Develop.

The Leaves of the Plants are designed to Transform the Un-Seen Energy of the Sun into a Chemical form that we can Digest to 'un-lock' and use it. They manifest a Seen physical form so that we may Eat The SUN !!!

The Energy from the Sun IS our Life Energy. Our Cells need Oxygen and Glucose (Sun Energy) for Growth and Development.

The Roots of the Plants are designed to Extract the Un-Seen Energy from the Earth, so that the Plant can Transform it into a Chemical form (Vitamins and Minerals), so that we can Digest and Extract the Energy from the Plants.

We Come from the Earth. The Vitamins and Minerals that we need to replenish and maintain Self = Hair, Nails and Skin, are found IN the Fruits and Veggies on the Earth = HUMAN FOOD!!!!!

THER IS NO LIFE ENERGY PRESENT IM ANIMAL MEATS !!!!!!!!!

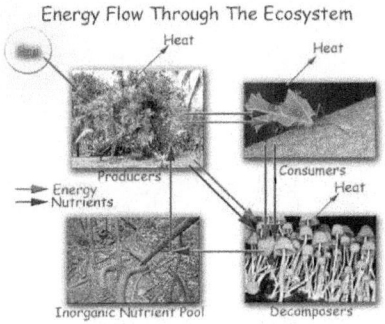
Energy Flow Through The Ecosystem

Ecology: Energy Flow and Nutrient Cycles

Essential Questions:

How does Energy Flow through the Earth?

How do Nutrients Cycle through the Earth?

How are these processes related to each other to sustain life on Earth?

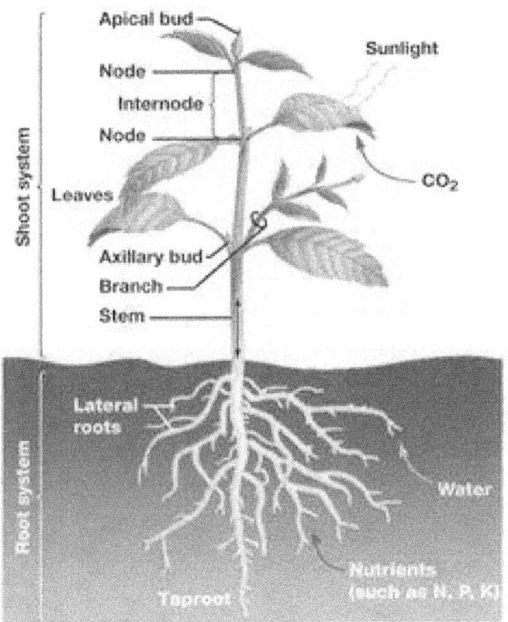

Critical thinking

- Draw an energy pyramid for a five-step food chain. If 100 percent of the energy is available at the first trophic level, what is the percentage of the total energy is available at the **highest** trophic level

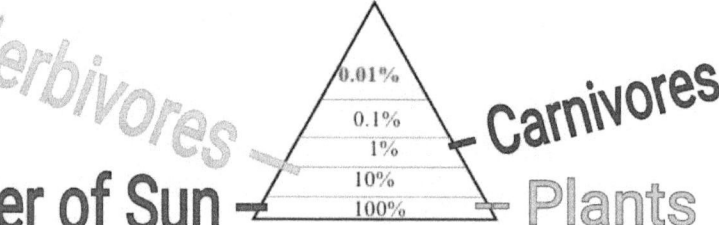

*****

Chapter Ten .... The Trophic/Energy Levels

*****

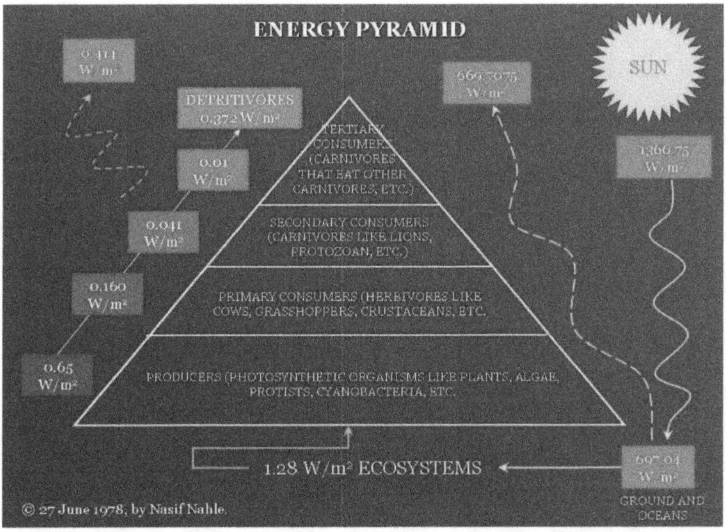

Trophic Levels is the Bio-availability of Energy between and for the classes of eaters, which are Herbivores, Carnivores, Omnivores and Scavengers. The Sun (along with the Earth and Water) provides the Energy that is available within our Eco-System.

Energy cannot be destroyed, only transformed and/or transferred into another state. The Life Energy of the Sun is transferred in Plants (Fruits and Veggies), and through the action of Photosynthesis, is transformed into the Chemical form Glucose (as well as other Nutrients that support the Metabolizing of the Life Energy).

The circle below represents the producer. All of the Stored Life Energy present in the body of the Producer Organism / Plant that is eaten by the Primary Consumer / Herbivore:

Without the Organisms capable of producing our Life Energy, there would be no way for the any of the Life Forms on Earth to sustain themselves. Plants and other Primary Producers manifest the Life Energy that we consume and dispense for us the Oxygen that we Breathe. This process is essential for continuation of our Life here on Earth.

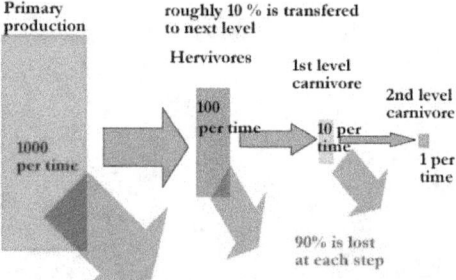

The Transfer of Energy in Food Chain!

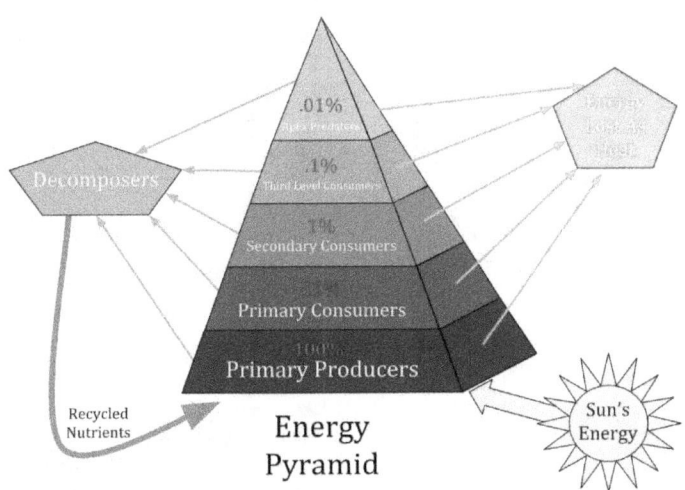

Energy
Pyramid

When we Herbivores eat the Naturally occurring Fruits and Veggies we are taking Natural Life Energy into our Bodies. We can represent the amount of energy taken in by a herbivore *the* as an energy circle.

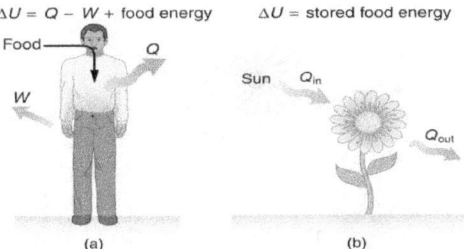

As Herbivores, we will use this energy for movement and other body activities, such as reproduction and movement. Some parts of the plant which was eaten cannot be digested by the herbivore; the energy in these parts of the plant passes out of the herbivore's body as waste.

Some of the energy, however, is used for growth and remains as organic matter in the herbivore's body. It is this energy which can be eaten by the secondary consumer.

The circle below represents the primary consumer. Only the stored energy is eaten by the secondary consumer:

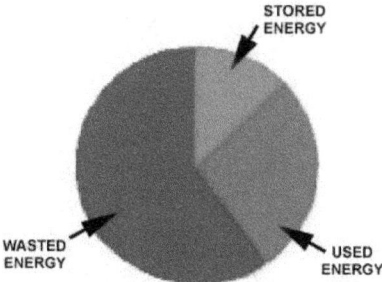

As you can see from the diagrams (left), only about 10% of the energy which the plant used for growth is taken into the body of the carnivore. The second consumer uses some of this energy for its own body activities and some of the energy will be wasted. Therefore, the amount of energy available for the tertiary consumer is only 1% of the energy which the primary consumer gained from the plant.

As the Life Energy is passed along our Bio-Food Chain a majority of it is either Used or Lost. Therefore, there is a limit to the number of Organisms/Consumers within a specific Bio-Food chain. The top Consumer/Carnivore is usually no more than the third or fourth Consumer where there is almost NO Life Energy left.

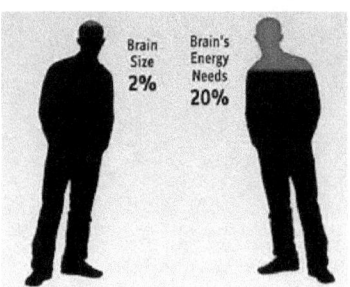

THIS MAKES HUMANS BEING PRIMARY CONSUMERS/HERBIVORES THAT MUCH MORE IMPORTANT. ESPECIALLY SINCE OUR BRAIN REQUIRES AT LEAST 20% OF OUR TOTAL ENERGY INTAKE FOR BASIC PERFORMANCE.

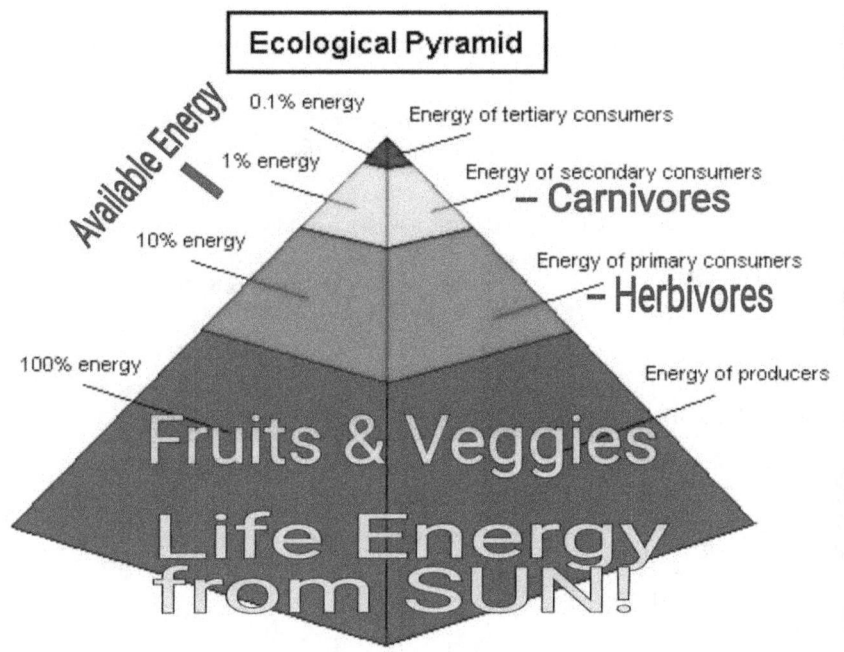

The circle below represents the secondary consumer. Only a very small fraction (shown in green) of the producer's original energy is stored by the secondary consumer. This energy is taken into the body of the tertiary consumer.

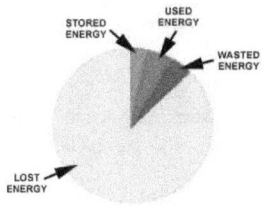

The Secondary Consumer is the Carnivore, and as the above diagram shows, there is LESS than Half the Bio-Available Life Energy that is present in animal meats (this amount is subject to conditions of slaughter, storage and cooking methods).

Carnivores consume their meat RAW and without breads or side-items or condiments. The Bio-available Life Energy in animal meats is IN the Blood – NOT the fabric of the flesh.

Carnivores have a very short Digestive Tract, which allows them to extract the Nutrients and quickly discard the undigested flesh, BEFORE it can rot and ferment INSIDE of it.

THE ENERGY CARNOVORES EXTRACT FROM FLESH IS THE REMAINING 1% BIO-AVAILABLE ENERGY FROM THE PRIMARY PRODUCERS.

SO, Carnivores eat flesh to Extract the SAME Life Energy the Herbivores eat = Primary Producers = Fruits & Veggies!

So, HOW can a claim of ANY vital Nutrients being necessary for our growth and development manifest from such a SMALL amount of Bio-available Life Energy ?

Especially when animal flesh is hard for Humans to Digest!

Table of Food and Liquid Transit Time (to Exit the Stomach)	
Water (Aspirin, Alcohol)	0-10 Minutes
Juice	15-30 Minutes
Fruit	30-60 Minutes
Melons	30-60 Minutes
Sprouts	1 Hour
Wheatgrass Juice	60-90 Minutes
Most Vegetables	1-2 Hours
Grains and Beans	1-2 Hours
Dense Vegetable Protein (Nuts, Seeds, Avocados)	2-3 Hours
Cooked Meat and Fish	3-4 Hours
Shellfish	4-8 Hours
Any Improperly Combined Meal	8 Hours

Animal flesh has the greatest amount of Digestion time because it is NOT Human food.

Digestion of food requires Energy. The premise is that our Bodies receive MORE Energy from the food than it expended to Digest it. This is our Energy cycle.

We Humans represent the Primary Consumers - which are Herbivores. Herbivores are the most Powerful and Intelligent of all the Consumers because they receive the maximum LIFE Energy available. They eat directly and only from the Producers. They Eat the SUN !!

CORRECT FOOD COMBINING QUICK REFERENCE CHART

	Protein	Starch	Fat	Sweet Milk	Sour Milk	Starchy Vegetables	Non-starchy Green Vegetables	Acid Fruits	Sub-acid Fruits	Sweet fruits (dried)	Melons
Protein - Flesh	bad	bad	bad	bad	bad	bad	good	bad	bad	bad	bad
Protein - Fat (nuts)	bad	bad	bad	bad	bad	bad	good	good	bad	bad	bad
Protein - Starch	bad	fair	fair	bad	bad	good	good	bad	bad	bad	bad
Starch	bad	good	good	bad	bad	good	good	bad	bad	bad	bad
Fat	bad	good	good	fair	fair	good	good	fair	bad	bad	bad
Sweet Milk	bad	bad	good			bad	bad	fair	fair	bad	bad
Sour Milk	bad	bad	good			bad	bad	fair	fair	bad	bad
Green Vegetables†	good	good	good	poor	bad	good	good	good	fair	poor	bad
Sub-acid Fruits†	bad	bad	good	fair	fair	bad	fair	good	good	good	bad
Acid Fruits	bad*	bad	good*	fair	fair	bad	fair	good	good	bad	fair
Sweet Fruits‡	bad	bad	bad	poor	fair	bad	poor	poor	good	good	bad
Melons	bad	bad	bad	bad	bad	bad	bad	fair	bad	bad	good

*Acid fruits are Fair with Nuts.   †Raw or cooked   ‡Dried   Avocados are Fair with Starch & Bad with Protein.
Tomatoes: Don't combine with ANY form of Proteins, except Nuts & Acid Fruits.

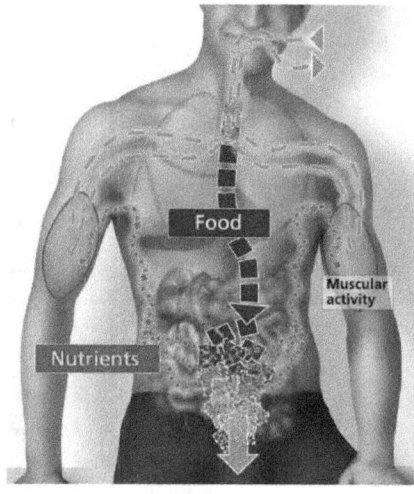

When food, which contains Stored Chemical Energy is taken into the body, it undergoes several changes that convert it into different Storage forms of Chemical Energy. This Chemical Energy is then available to be used and converted further as Work is performed.

Chemical Energy is transformed in to Mechanical Energy when our Muscles contract.

Chemical Energy is transformed into Thermal Energy in the regulation and control of our Body Temperature.

Chemical Energy is needed to build new Tissues and Molecules for growth and Metabolism. Throughout all of this Work, Heat is manifested off into the surrounding Atmosphere and onto larger Biosphere.

In the human body energy is present as either *Free Energy* or *Potential Energy*. Free energy is the energy being used at any given moment in the performance of a task. It is unbound and in motion. Potential energy is energy that is stored or bound in a chemical compound and can be converted to free energy when needed.

For example, the energy stored in carbohydrate is potential energy. When we eat carbohydrate and it is metabolized, energy is released for body work. As work is completed, this energy, now in the form of heat or thermal energy, is given off into the air. Measurement of the amount of heat produced over time makes it possible for us to express body energy consumption in kilocalories (kcalories or kcal) or units of heat.

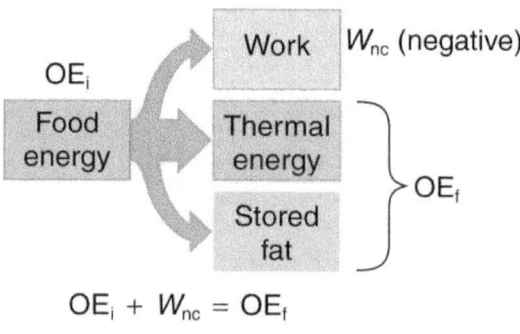

$$OE_i + W_{nc} = OE_f$$

All foods that provides Energy is measured in units called KCalories (commonly referred to as Calories).

Calories are taken into our bodies as carbohydrates, proteins, and fats (which are known as macronutrients, or major constituents of diet). We also require vitamins and minerals (which are effective in small amounts and thus are known as micronutrients) to process these nutrients and maintain body functions.

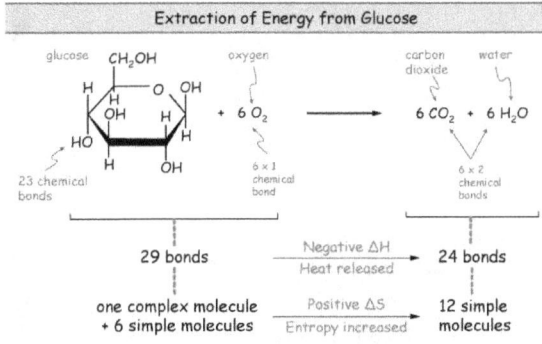

The Energy Manifested in the form of Kcals isn't necessarily the same as LIFE Energy. Our Cells need OXYGEN and GLUCOSE for growth and development.

Our Brains specifically NEED GLUCOSE.

ONLY CARBOHYDRATES MANIFEST OUR LIFE ENERGY IN THE FORM OF GLUCOSE!

Nutritionists generally recommend daily intake of 1600 calories for older adults and sedentary women; 2200 calories for children, teenage girls, active women, and sedentary men; and 2800 calories for teenage boys, active men, and very active women.

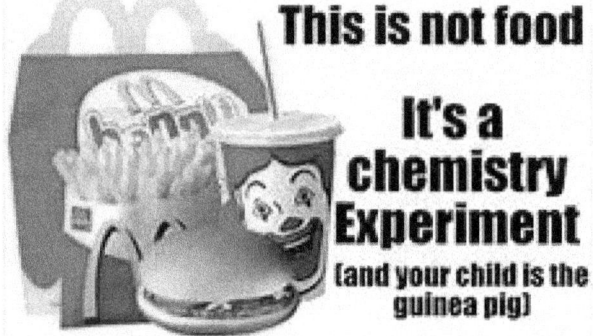

COSMETIC CHEMICALS IN FAST FOOD?!

Sodium Stearoyl Lactylate
Found in shampoo and soap
Reasoning for use: 'dough
conditioner' even though bread does
not require this, and has been made
without SSL for thousands of years

Calcium Disodium EDTA
Found in skin products and hair
conditioner (used as stabilizer)
Reasoning for use: Flavor protectant
in fast food sauces, dips and
dressings

Ammonium Glycyrrhizin
Found in facial mask products
Reasoning for use: Flavor
enhancer, flavoring agent, surface-

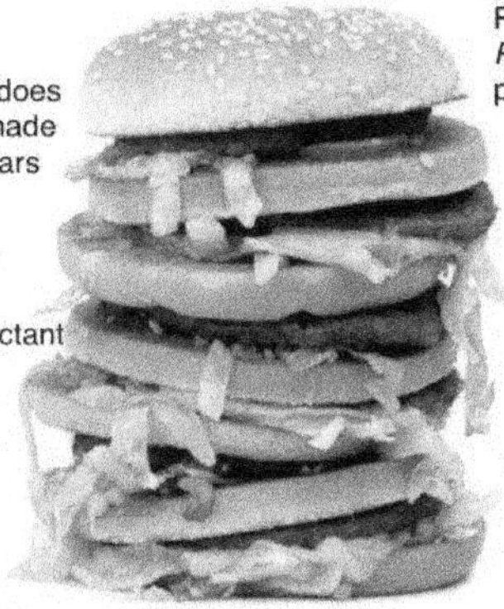

Disodium Phosphate
Found in mascara and mouthwash
Reasoning for use: Food
preservative

Propylene Glycol
Found in shampoo, mouthwash,
hand sanitizers
Reasoning for use: Gives most of
today's food and beverages their
distinctive taste

Benzoyl Peroxide
*Recently banned in China
Active ingredient in acne creams
Reasoning for use: Bleaching wheat
flour white (all fast food breads)

******

Chapter Eleven…. YOU ARE WHAT YOU EAT

*****

HUMAN GENOME
~25,000 genes
packaged in every
human cell

A cell

Chromosomes – 23 pairs

The chromosome is
made up of genes

The genes consist of DNA
which is made up of four
chemical letters

EPIGENETICS:

Environment (temperature,
radiation, food, drugs,
nutrients produce
immediate effects that can
be imprinted long-term

MUTATION HERE CAN
PRODUCE GENOTYPES OR
RARE GENETIC DISORDERS

The Human Body is a by-product of the Earth and every part of ourselves has a direct symbiotic relationship with parts of the Earth.

To be considered Healthy, our Body needs to be replenished with the Earth that it came from. This is the purpose and function of Fruits and Veggies. The Un-Seen Energy from the Sun and Earth is perfectly manifested in the Chemical (Seen) form that is referred to as Nutrients.

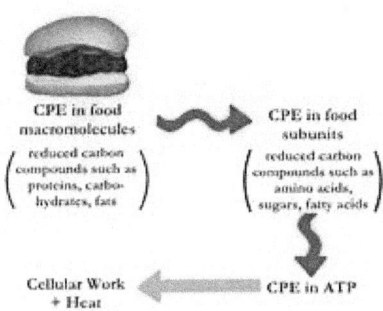

CPE in food
macromolecules

reduced carbon
compounds such as
proteins, carbo-
hydrates, fats

CPE in food
subunits

reduced carbon
compounds such as
amino acids,
sugars, fatty acids

Cellular Work
+ Heat

CPE in ATP

During Digestion, the Molecular structure of the food is transformed, and the Bonds are broken and Life Energy released. Of the elements that are listed as Nutrients, it's the Macro-Nutrients that yield or release Life Energy, particularly Carbohydrates, specifically in the form of Glucose. Lipids or Fats would be considered an emergency or secondary Life Energy source, because in the absence of Carbs can be used to Synthesize Life Energy.

Protein is also a Macro-Nutrient that in an Emergency or Carb and Fat deficient environment by used to Synthesize Glucose and provide Life Energy

There is NO Life Energy in the Chemical form of Glucose or Carbohydrates presented in the Digestion of ANY Animal Meats.

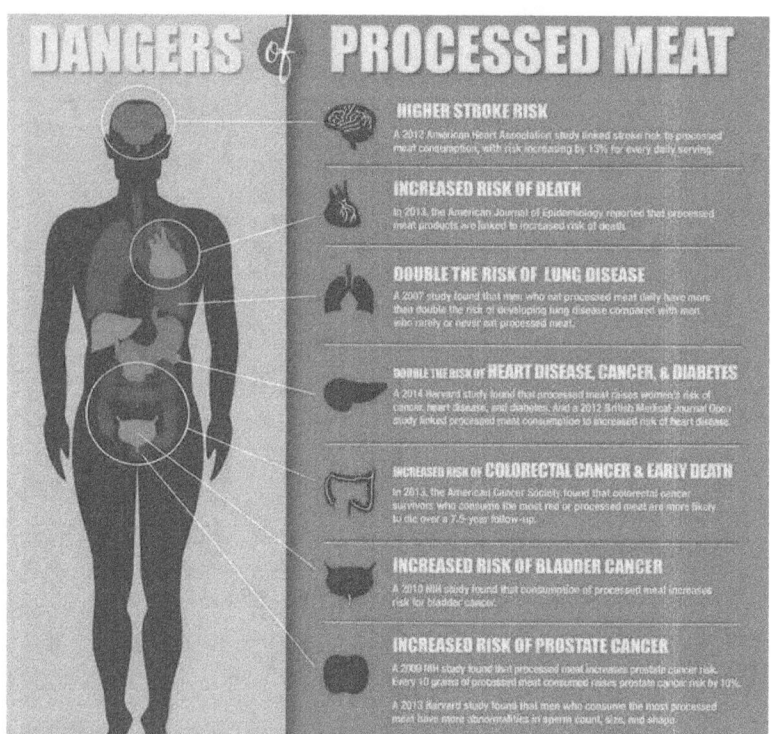

Animal meats do manifest Macro-Nutrients in the form of Protein and Fat, however they also present potentially Toxic levels of 'Bad' Cholesterol. The Lipids/Fats that they release is the Saturated or 'Bad' Lipids.

In this day in age, most animals are raised in mass production, fed a variety of growth hormones, steroids, anti-biotics, and several other TOXIC medications to produce the desired meat or egg production. And their living conditions are usually deplorable, unsanitary and ripe with dangerous bacteria and Viruses. Add to this the TERROR filled way that most are slaughtered – which releases the Chemical Hormones of FEAR into Fabric of Meat, makes ALL animal meats that much more TOXIC!

The Characteristics of WHAT you eat is incorporated and assimilated INTO self. No matter HOW much Protein of Vitamin B12 is proposed to be in the Cow/Beef, Cows are Slow moving, Easily Led to Slaughter, Fearful, Docile animal, that when consumed = *You ARE What You EAT!*

There is no Life Energy manifested from consuming Chickens. The Protein that they possess is DENATURED during the 'cooking' process and transformed into a Chemical Composition of Protein that our Bodies CANNOT utilize. Chickens also possess such a FEARFUL Nature that a Human that displays Fear is referred to as a 'chicken'. The Mating ritual between a Rooster and Hen is VIOLENT - the Rooster STANDS on the Back of the Hen and pulls on the back of her neck with his beak, making

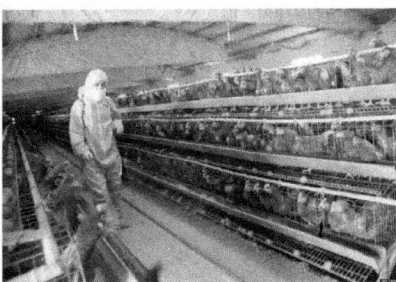

her cry out in pain and submit. And chickens are CANNIBALS... they do eat their own Eggs. Chickens are also some of the most Selfish animals on Earth, as well as great Scavengers and will eat anything they can swallow = *You ARE What You EAT!*

MEAT AND CANCER
HOW STRONG IS THE EVIDENCE?

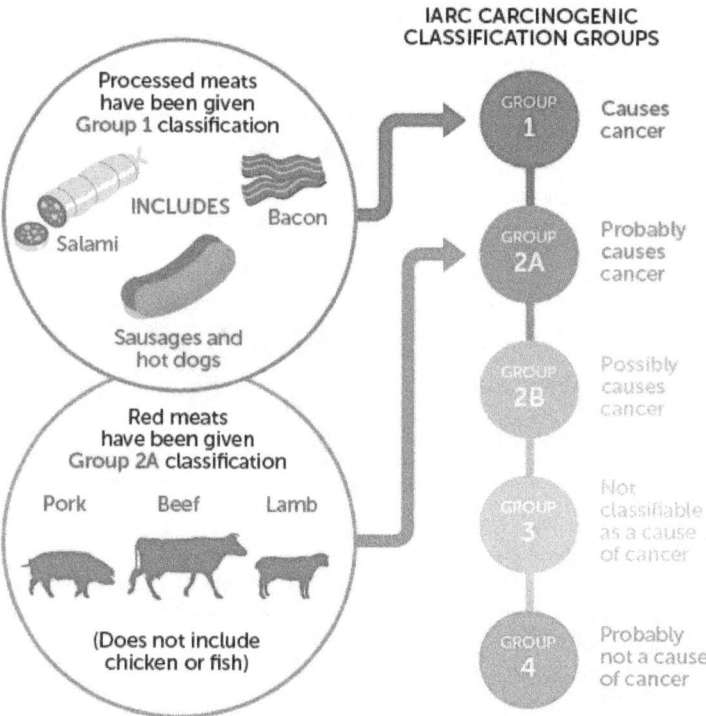

IARC CARCINOGENIC CLASSIFICATION GROUPS

Processed meats have been given Group 1 classification

INCLUDES

Salami — Bacon

Sausages and hot dogs

Red meats have been given Group 2A classification

Pork   Beef   Lamb

(Does not include chicken or fish)

GROUP 1 — Causes cancer

GROUP 2A — Probably causes cancer

GROUP 2B — Possibly causes cancer

GROUP 3 — Not classifiable as a cause of cancer

GROUP 4 — Probably not a cause of cancer

These categories represent how likely something is to cause cancer in humans, not how many cancers it causes.

Regardless of your spiritual beliefs, there may be good reason to carefully consider your decision to include pork as a regular part of your diet, because despite advertising campaigns trying to paint pork as a "healthy" alternative to beef, research suggests it may be hazardous to your health on multiple levels.

MEAT—ANY MEAT—COSTS LIVES.

"It promotes intolerable suffering and disease—not only among animals, but also for many Americans by raising their risk of HEART DISEASE, DIABETES, BREAST CANCER, and EARLY DEATH."

- Neal Barnard, M.D.

One of the most potentially acute hazards is contamination with pathogenic bacteria.

According to a surprising new investigation by *Consumer Reports*[1], 69 percent of all raw pork samples tested — nearly 200 samples in total — were contaminated with the dangerous bacteria Yersinia enterocolitica, which causes fever and gastrointestinal illness with diarrhea, vomiting, and stomach cramps.

Ground pork was more likely than pork chops to be contaminated.

The pork also tested positive for other contaminants, including the controversial drug ractopamine, which is banned in many parts of the world, including China and Europe. The drug, which was found in more than 20 percent of the samples, is used to boost growth in the animal while leaving the meat lean. Worst of all, many of the bacteria found in the pork were resistant to multiple antibiotics, making treatment, should you fall ill, all the more problematic and potentially lethal.

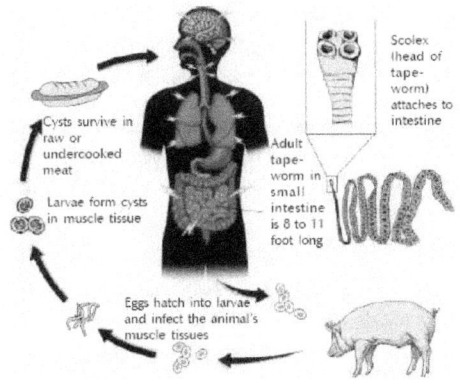

Cysts survive in raw or undercooked meat

Larvae form cysts in muscle tissue

Eggs hatch into larvae and infect the animal's muscle tissues

Egg contaminated vegetation is ingested by livestock

Scolex (head of tapeworm) attaches to intestine

Adult tapeworm in small intestine is 8 to 11 foot long

According to the featured report:

"We found salmonella, staphylococcus aureus, or listeria monocytogenes, more common causes of foodborne illness, in 3 to 7 percent of samples. And 11 percent harbored enterococcus, which can indicate fecal contamination and can cause problems such as urinary-tract infections."

Nearly all pigs raised in the U.S. come from Concentrated Animal Feeding Operations, or CAFO's. These inhumane environments are typically toxic breeding grounds for pathogens.

These animals spend their short, miserable lives on concrete and steel grates. Antibiotics are given liberally with their feed, making their massive waste even more toxic.

This is why you can smell a CAFO swine operation miles before you see it. At an operation like Joel Salatin's, you couldn't smell any sign of pigs. These pigs were raised humanely and organically, where both animal and land are managed symbiotically.

Unfortunately, raising animals in CAFO's is the standard for Americans. For many of us, CAFO pork is the only option available.

Bacon's Cancer Risk

How much bacon you have to eat to raise your risk of colorectal cancer

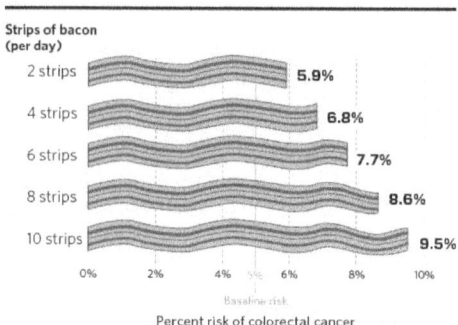

This is why my Nutrition Plan recommends consciously avoiding pork whenever possible unless you can assure yourself that the hogs were raised like the video above. Eating Pork and it's by-products is a risk, and the more you consume it the more likely it is that you will eventually acquire some type of infection. The pork and swine industry has been continually plagued, and continues to be so to this day, by a wide variety of hazardous infections and diseases, including:

- **PRRS** -- A horrendous disease, which I first reported on in 2001, but which had been a nightmare for many nations since the mid-1980s, is still alive and kicking today. At one point referred to as "swine mystery disease," "blue abortion," and "swine infertility," the disease was finally named "Porcine Reproductive and Respiratory Syndrome" (PRRS), and may afflict about 75 percent of American pig herds.

The PRRS virus primarily attacks the pig's immune system, leaving its body open to a host of infections, particularly in the lungs. Initial research revealed that the virus was transmitted via semen, saliva and blood, leaving pigs herded closely together and transported in close quarters by trucks more susceptible to infection. However, according to research presented at the 2007 International PRRS Symposium, the disease is also airborne, making eradication efforts very difficult.

- **The Nipah Virus** - Discovered in 1999, the Nipah virus has caused disease in both animals and humans, through contact with infected animals. In humans, the virus can lead to deadly encephalitis (an acute inflammation of your brain). I originally reported on this virus in 2000, but according to CDC data, the Nipah virus reemerged again in 2004.

- **Porcine Endogenous Retrovirus (PERV)** - According to a study in the journal Lancet, this virus can spread to people receiving pig organ transplants, and according to test tube studies, PERV strains do have the ability to infect human cells.

- PERV genes are scattered throughout pigs' genetic material, and researchers have found that pig heart, spleen and kidney cells release various strains of the virus.

- **Menangle Virus** – In 1998, it was reported that a new virus infecting pigs was able to jump to humans. The menangle virus was discovered in August 1997 when sows at an Australian piggery began giving birth to deformed and mummified piglets.

Pork is NOT Advisable in a Raw Diet

As explained by *Consumer Reports*, thoroughly cooking your pork is important for safety, so if you're on a raw diet (which can include raw meats), pork should definitely NOT be part of your menu... Again, while I don't recommend it, if you DO opt to eat pork, it would be wise to follow these safe handling tips and guidelines, issued by *Consumer Reports*[1]:

- *When cooking pork, use a meat thermometer to ensure that it reaches the proper internal temperature, which kills potentially harmful bacteria: at least 145° F for whole pork and 160° F for ground pork.*

- *Keep raw pork and its juices separate from other foods, especially those eaten raw, such as salad.*

- *Wash your hands thoroughly after handling raw meat.*

- *Choose pork and other meat products that were raised without drugs. One way to do that is to buy certified organic pork, from pigs raised without antibiotics or ractopamine.*

- *Look for a clear statement regarding antibiotic use. "No antibiotics used" claims with a USDA Process Verified shield are more reliable than those without verification. Labels such as "Animal Welfare Approved" and "Certified Humane" indicate the prudent use of antibiotics to treat illness.*

- *Watch out for misleading labels. "Natural" has nothing to do with antibiotic use or how an animal was raised. We found unapproved claims, including "no antibiotic residues," on packages of Sprouts pork sold in California and Arizona, and "no antibiotic growth promotants" on Farmland brand pork sold in several states. We reported those to the USDA in June 2012, and the agency told us it's working with those companies to take "appropriate actions." When we checked in early November, Sprouts had removed the claim from its packages.*

- *If your local supermarket doesn't carry pork from pigs raised without antibiotics, consider asking the store to carry it. To find meat from animals that were raised sustainably – humanely and without drugs – go to eatwellguide.org. To learn about the Consumers Union campaign aimed at getting stores to sell only antibiotic-free meat, go to NotinMyFood.org.*

WHO classification of red and processed meats

IARC* Carcinogenic Classification Groups

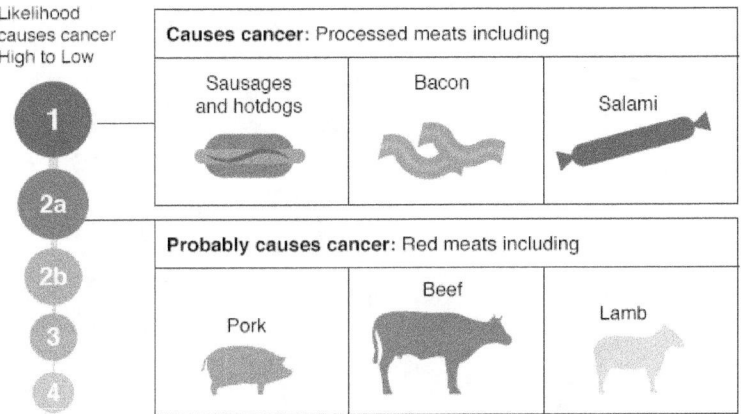

Likelihood causes cancer High to Low

Causes cancer: Processed meats including

| Sausages and hotdogs | Bacon | Salami |

Probably causes cancer: Red meats including

| Pork | Beef | Lamb |

Source: Cancer Research UK, WHO   *International Agency for Research on Cancer   BBC

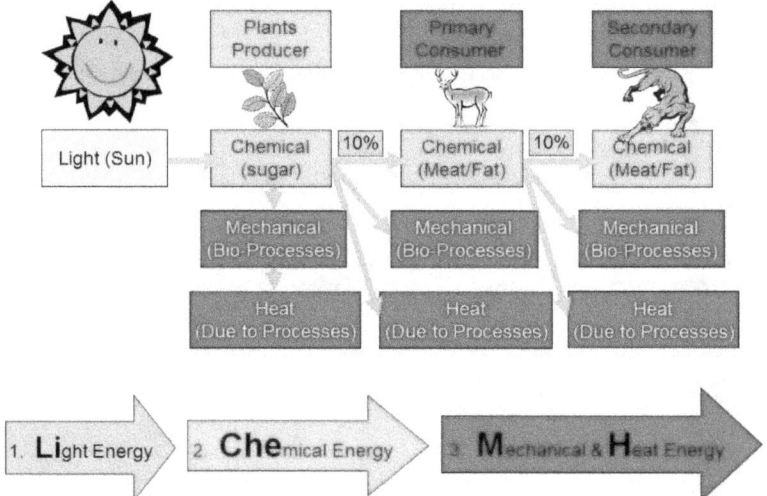

*****

Chapter Twelve.... Understanding Glucose

*****

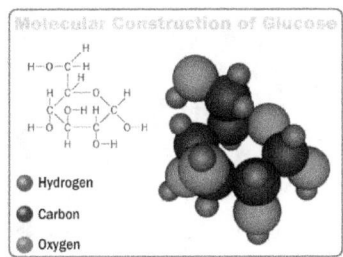

The carbohydrate glucose is very important substance in biology and in metabolism of all life forms. Glucose is a simple sugar, or monosaccharide, and is the main and preferred source of energy for red blood cells, the brain and the nervous system.

Glucose also plays a role in the creation or synthesis of other substances like glycoproteins or glycolipids. It can create or synthesize polysaccharides, which are complex sugars that can be used as energy storage in organisms as well.

Glucose is a component of a variety of carbohydrates in the body. It can form disaccharides like sucrose, which is also known as table sugar, or lactose, which is the sugar found in milk, according to the book "Nutrition."

Glucose can also form polysaccharides, such as glycogen, which is a form of energy storage. When the amount of glucose exceeds the amount of energy needed by the body, the extra glucose is converted into glycogen and stored in the liver. When the body's energy needs increasing, the glycogen is changed back into glucose.

Your body can break down fats and even proteins to get the energy it needs. But it's glucose, derived from the digestion of carbohydrates, that your body desires. Glucose is the main source of energy for every single cell, and it is the preferred energy type for brain cells. If you have diabetes, your body has problems handling glucose, which can be very dangerous for your health.

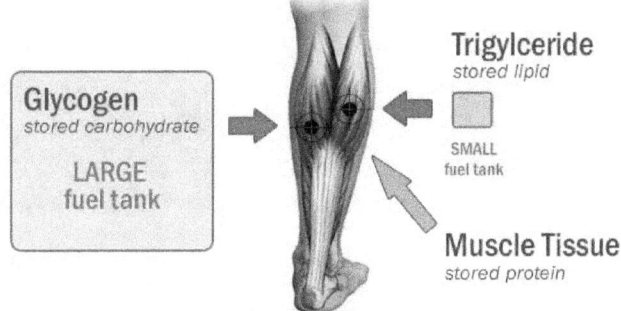

Glucose Conversion

All Carbohydrates, with the exception of Fiber, eventually wind up metabolized as Glucose – our primary source of Energy = Life Energy.

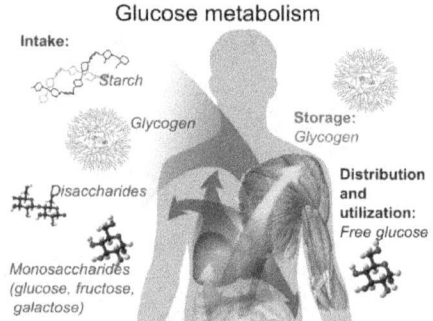

Glucose metabolism

However, the way they get there varies. Sugars, which are Simple Carbs, are very small Molecules that convert into Glucose quickly after combining with Enzymes in your Small Intestine.

Starches, which are Complex Carbohydrates, undergo numerous steps before Glucose is formed. When you chew, your mouth secretes Saliva, an Enzyme that starts breaking down Complex Starch compounds. Saliva turns Starches into a kind of Simple Carbohydrate.

As the Simple Molecules approach your Small Intestine, the Enzymes there kick in again to break them down further, converting them into Glucose.

Glucose can also play a role in the creation of non-Carbohydrate molecules as well. Glucose is part of the pathway that creates the building blocks for either DNA or RNA, according to Chronolab.com.

According to EdInformatics.com, Glucose is vital to the production of Proteins and Lipids, and may help theses Proteins or Lipids assume it's appropriate folded shape. Glucose also plays a role in the production of Vitamin C.

Cellular Respiration: Energy for Life

Life Energy

To start the process of Pellular Respiration, we need to get glucose into our cells. The first step is to eat a Carbohydrate-rich food, made of Glucose.

Let's say we eat a Apple. That Apple travels through our Digestive System, where it is broken down and absorbed into the Blood.

The Glucose then travels to our Cells, where it is let inside.

Once inside, the cells use various **Enzymes**, or small Proteins that speed up c\Chemical reactions, to change Glucose into different Molecules.

The goal of this process is to release the Life Energy stored in the Bonds of Atoms that make up Glucose.

① Glycolysis, which takes place in the cytosol, splits glucose, a six-carbon molecule, into two three-carbon molecules (pyruvate). This step releases high-energy electrons (purple balls) and produces a small amount of ATP. Pyruvate is then either broken down to produce more ATP or is used to remake glucose.

② Pyruvate can be used to produce more ATP when oxygen is available. In the mitochondria, pyruvate is broken down, releasing carbon dioxide (CO_2) and high-energy electrons and forming acetyl-CoA (2 carbons), which continues through aerobic metabolism.

Let's examine each of the steps in Cellular Respiration next.

③ Acetyl-CoA enters the citric acid cycle, where carbon dioxide and high-energy electrons are released and where a small amount of ATP is produced.

④ Most ATP is produced in the final step of aerobic metabolism. Here the energy in the high-energy electrons released in previous steps is transferred to ATP, and the electrons are combined with oxygen and hydrogen to form water.

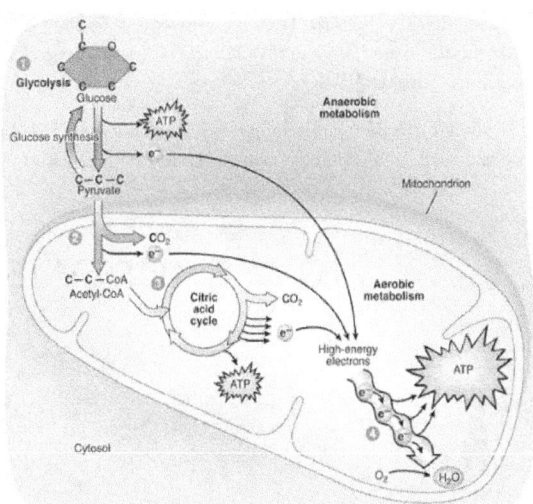

Steps of Cellular Respiration: Creating Life Energy

There are three steps of cellular respiration: glycolysis, the citric acid cycle, and oxidative phosphorylation. The main role of glucose in each of these steps is to provide energy in its bonds.

Step 1: Glycolysis

In glycolysis, glucose enters the cell. Next, a series of enzymes convert it to a different form called pyruvate in the main compartment of the cell, the cytoplasm. Two pyruvate are formed from one glucose. During this process two ATP are formed, as are two more of another energy-rich molecule called NADH. NADH collects electrons from the bonds in glucose. It transports them to the last step, oxidative phosphorylation, where they will be used to make ATP. So, the end purpose of glycolysis is to get a little ATP and harvest electrons in the bonds of glucose.

Step 2: Citric Acid Cycle

In the citric acid cycle, the pyruvate is converted to another molecule called acetyl Co-A. Acetyl Co-A undergoes a similar sequence of conversions to harvest more electrons in the form of NADH and make two ATP. These steps occur in the powerhouse of the cell, the mitochondria.

Step 3: Oxidative Phosphorylation

In the last step, all of the electrons harvested in the form of NADH from Glucose are transported to the Membrane of the Mitochondria. Here these Electrons are used by Proteins in our Cells to ultimately convert the Energy stored in them to ATP. In doing this, Oxygen combines with the Electrons and Hydrogen Ions to make Water.

Without Oxygen – the Breath Of Life, the Glucose – Life Energy, would be useless, and the chain of reactions in Cellular Respiration would get backed up and stop = pre-mature death.

How energy is released.

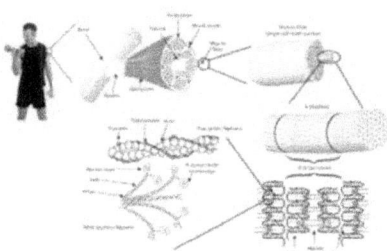

When you need energy, cells release chemical energy from glucose. You need food energy to run, walk and even sleep. Your cells use energy from food to carry out all of their activities.

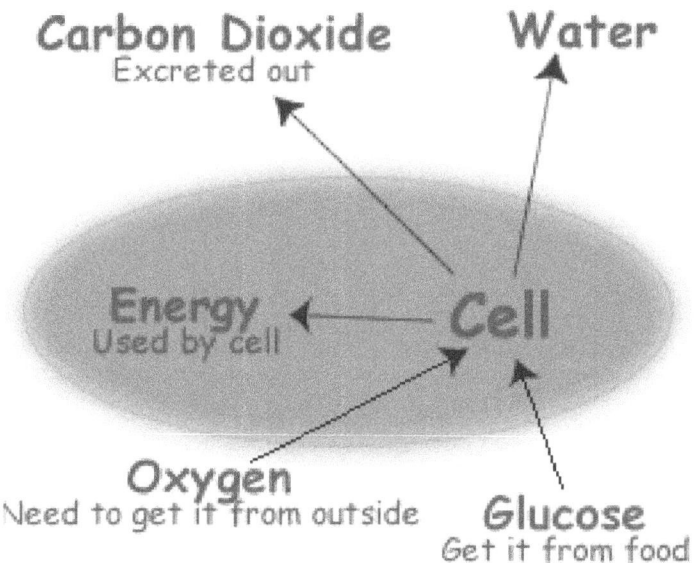

*****

Chapter Thirteen .... Importance of Glucose

*****

Every Cell of our Human body requires Energy to perform the Metabolic functions that sustain Life. Glucose is a small, Simple Sugar that serves as a primary fuel for our Energy production, especially for the Brain, Muscles and several other body Organs and Tissues.

Glucose also serves as a building block for larger structural Molecules of the body, such as Glycoproteins and Gycolipids. Our Human body tightly regulates Glucose levels. Abnormally high or low levels result in serious, potentially life-threatening complications.

Brain Fuel

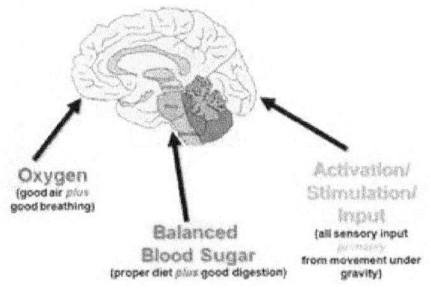

Oxygen
(good air *plus*
good breathing)

**Balanced
Blood Sugar**
(proper diet *plus* good digestion)

**Activation/
Stimulation/
Input**
(all sensory input
primarily
from movement under
gravity)

Our Brain relies exclusively on Glucose to create the fuel its transforms into its Energy needs. Because our Brain is responsible for the high-energy output of producing THOUGHT, it has a high-energy demand.

Because the Brain cannot store Glucose, the brain requires a constant and quality supply of the Life Energy. Our body possesses multiple mechanisms to prevent a significant drop in our Blood Glucose supply, known as Hypoglycemia by producing what we call 'CRAVINGS' to make us aware of being Energy Deficient so we can eat.

Now, should such a drop occur, however, Brain functions can begin to IMMEDIATELY fail. Common Brain-related symptoms of Hypoglycemia (Low LIFE Energy) include headache, dizziness, confusion, lack of concentration, anxiety, irritability, restlessness, slurred speech and poor coordination. A sudden, severe drop on blood glucose can lead to seizures and coma.

Muscle Fuel

The skeletal muscles normally constitute approximately 30 to 40 percent of total body weight, although this varies based on sex, age and fitness level. Our Skeletal Muscles utilize large amounts of Glucose during exercise.

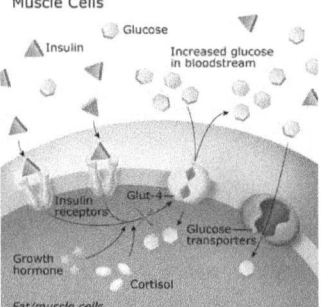

Glucose Counter-regulatory Hormones: Effect on Fat and Muscle Cells

Unlike our Brain, our Skeletal Muscles store Blood Sugar in the form of Glycogen, which is quickly broken down to supply Glucose during physical exertion. Muscle Tissue also normally absorbs large amounts of Glucose from the bloodstream during exercise.

Although skeletal muscles can utilize Fat-derived Molecules for Energy production, depletion of Glucose stores during prolonged exercise can lead to sudden fatigue -- commonly known as bonking or hitting the wall.

Fuel for Other Tissues and Organs

The various Organs and Tissues of the body have the capacity to utilize different fuels. In addition to the Brain and Skeletal muscles, some other important Organs and tissues also rely on glucose as their primary or sole fuel. Examples include the Cornea, Lens and Retina of the Eyes, and the Red and White Blood Cells. Interestingly, although the Cells of the Small Intestines are responsible for absorbing Glucose from food and passing it into the Bloodstream, they primarily use another Molecule called Glutamine for fuel. This leaves more Glucose for other Organs and Tissues that are more reliant on the Sugar.

Structural Roles

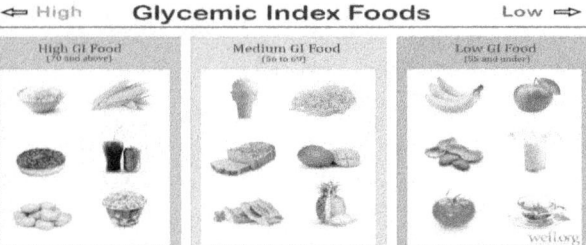

In addition to its role in Energy production, the Human body utilizes Glucose along with other substances to manufacture other important structural Molecules. For example, the Glycoprotein Collagen consists of a protein backbone plus simple sugars, including glucose.

Collagen is an essential structural molecule found in Skin, Muscles, Bones and other body Tissues. Other Glycoproteins play important roles in the development and maintenance of the Nerves of the Body.

Glycolipids, which consist of Fat and Sugar building blocks, are fundamental components of the Membranes that surround the individual Cells of the Body, as well as structures within these Cells.

Hypoglycemia and Hyperglycemia

A significant drop in blood sugar typically causes symptoms of hypoglycemia relatively quickly, because of the brain's exquisite dependence on a constant glucose supply.

A high Blood Glucose level, or Hyperglycemia, may or may not cause obvious symptoms. In people with type 1 diabetes, who have little to no production of the Blood-Sugar-lowering hormone Insulin, the combination of high Blood Sugar and lack of Insulin often leads to signs and symptoms, including:

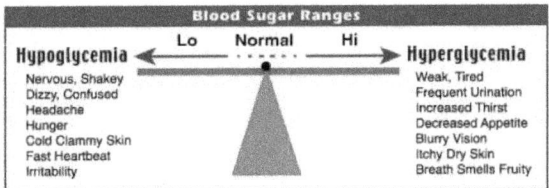

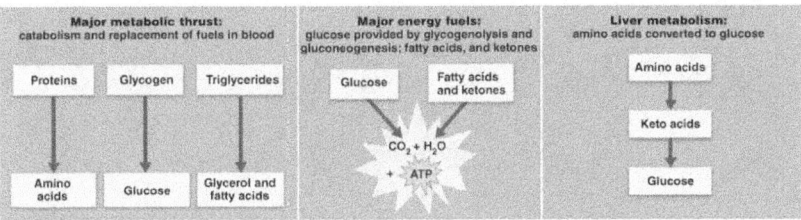

(a) Major events of the postabsorptive state

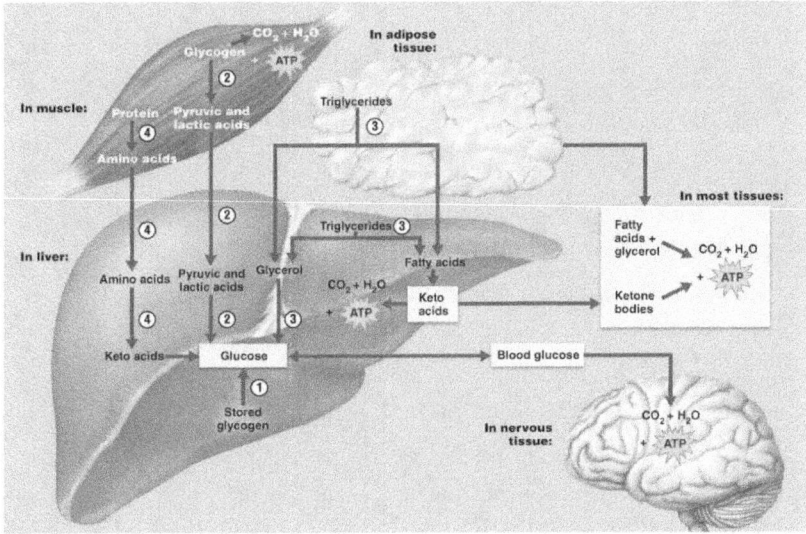

******

Chapter Fourteen.... Energy Balance: Input and Output!

******

TABLE 2.1   Estimated Energy Stores in Humans

Energy source	Storage site	Approximate energy (kcal)
ATP/CP*	Various tissues	5
Carbohydrate	Blood glucose	80
	Liver glycogen	400
	Muscle glycogen	1,500
Fat	Serum free fatty acids	7
	Serum triglycerides	75
	Muscle triglycerides	2,500
	Adipose tissue	80,000+
Protein	Muscle protein	30,000

*ATP/CP = adenosine triphosphate/creatine phosphate

We Humans, as well as other animals need a minimum intake of food Energy to sustain their Metabolism and to drive their Muscles.

Foods are composed chiefly of Carbohydrates, Fats, Proteins, Alcohol, Water, Vitamins, and Minerals. Carbohydrates, Fats, Proteins, Alcohol, and Water represent virtually all the weight of food, with Vitamins and Minerals making up only a small percentage of the weight.

(Carbohydrates, Fats, and Proteins comprise ninety percent of the dry weight of foods.) Organisms derive food Energy from Carbohydrates, Fats and Proteins as well as from organic Acids, Polyols, and Ethanol present in the diet.

Some diet components that provide little or no food Energy, such as Water, Minerals, Vitamins, Cholesterol, and Fiber, may still be necessary to health and survival for other reasons. Water, Minerals, Vitamins, and Cholesterol are not broken down (they are used by the body in the form in which they are absorbed) and so cannot be used for Energy.

Fiber, a type of Carbohydrate, cannot be completely digested by the human body. Ruminants can extract the food Energy from the Respiration of Cellulose because of Bacteria in their Rumens.

A constant supply of Energy is needed to sustain the activities essential to life, specifically to successfully achieve and maintain Homeostasis.

Energy is required to support internal needs along with the added expectations of physical activity.

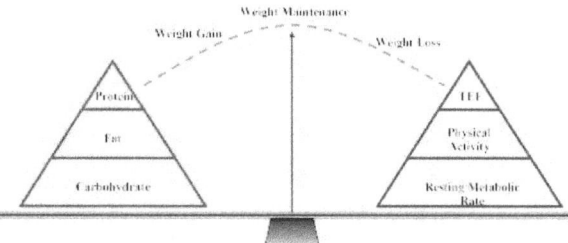

Whether the Energy used is Electrical, Mechanical, Thermal, or chemical, the supply of free Energy and the reservoir of Potential Energy decrease as the metabolic and physical work of the body continues; therefore, the system must be constantly refueled from an outside source.

For the Human Energy System, this outside fuel source is food.

Energy Control in Human Metabolism

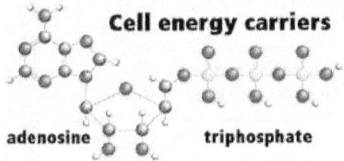

If the energy produced in the body through its many chemical reactions was "exploded" all at once, it would damage tissues and systems, so mechanisms are needed by which energy release can be controlled to support life, not destroy it. Two means of control make this possible: (1) **chemical bonding** and (2) controlled reaction rates.

Chemical Bonding

The primary mechanism controlling Energy release in the Human system is Chemical bonding.

The Chemical Bonds that hold elements together in compounds are our Life Energy Bonds. As long as the compound stays intact, Energy is being exerted to maintain it.

When the compound is broken into its parts, this Energy is released and becomes available for Work.

Bonds and Energy
- Energy is released when a bond forms
- Energy must be added to break a bond
- The amount of energy required to break a covalent bond is called the bond dissociation energy. It is always positive
- Endothermic Reaction- a greater amount of energy is required to break the existing bond in the reactants than is released
- Exothermic Reaction- more energy is released during product bond formation than is required to break bonds in the reactants.

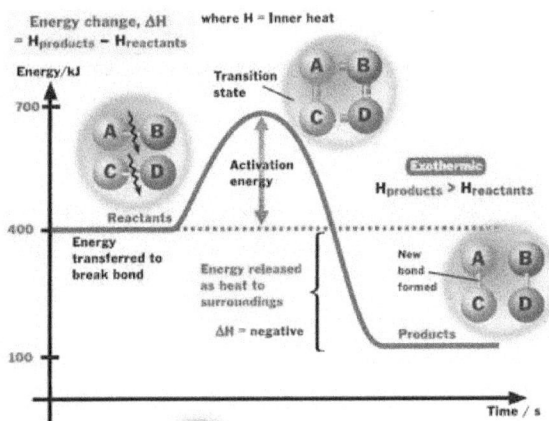

The following three types of Chemical Bonds transfer Energy:

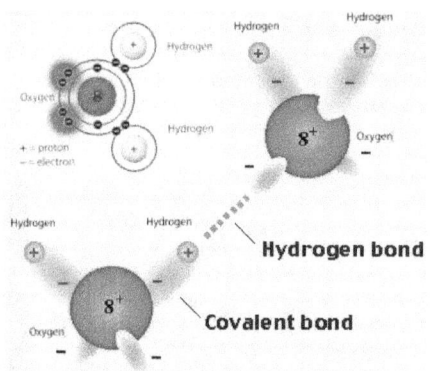

1. *Covalent bonds:* These bonds are based on the relative combining Power of the elements that make up a Compound. The Carbon Atoms in organic compounds such as Glucose are held together by Covalent Bonds.

2. *Hydrogen bonds:* Although weaker than Covalent Bonds, Hydrogen Bonds are significant because there are large numbers of them. In addition, the very fact that they are less strong and more easily broken allows them to transfer Energy readily from one substance to another. The Hydrogen attached to the Oxygen Molecule in the Carboxyl group (COOH-) of Amino Acids and Fatty Acids is an example of this type of Bond.

3. *High-Energy Phosphate bonds:* The High-Energy Phosphate Bonds in the compound **Adenosine Triphosphate (ATP)** are the major Energy source for carrying out our Body functions. Working like storage batteries for Electrical Energy, these Bonds are the controlling force of Energy Metabolism in the Human Cell.

ATP is Broken Down

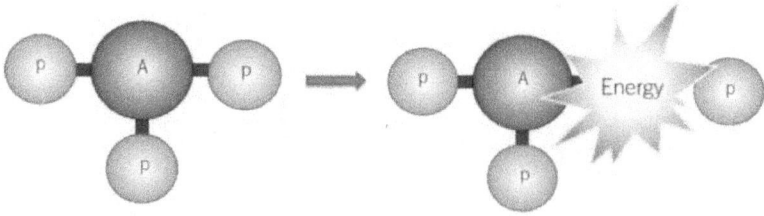

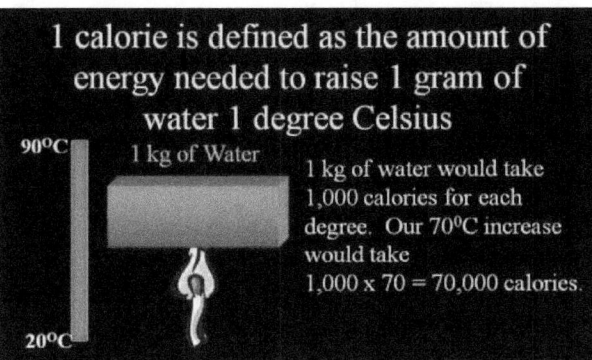

Measurement of Energy Balance

Kilocalorie

Because the release of energy and work performed by the Body produces Heat, Energy expenditure can be measured in Heat Equivalents. This measure of Heat is the **calorie**. To avoid having to calculate very large numbers, health professionals use the **kilocalorie** (KCalorie/Kcal) to describe Energy needs. The Kilocalorie is equal to 1000 Calories; this is the amount of heat required to raise 1 kg of water 1°C. (Materials prepared for the general public use the term *calorie*, although the actual measurement is the kilocalorie.)

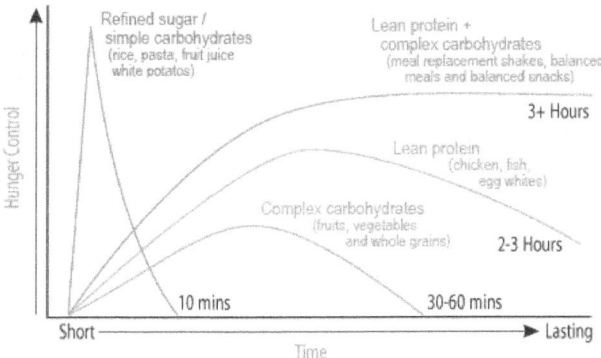

Food Energy Measurement

When helping people develop a food pattern appropriate to their Energy needs, it is necessary to know the Energy content of individual foods.

There are two methods for determining the Energy content of foods: (1) Direct **Calorimetry** or (2) calculation of approximate composition.

Calorimetry

The kcalorie values of foods given in food tables were determined by the method called *Direct Calorimetry.* This method uses a metal container called a *Bomb Calorimeter*, named from its long tubular shape.

A weighed amount of food is placed inside and the bomb calorimeter is immersed in water. The food is then ignited by an electric spark in the presence of Oxygen and burned to ash.

The increase in the temperature of the surrounding water indicates the number of kcalories given off by the complete oxidation of the food sample. When you use food tables, remember that these values represent averages from a number of samples of the given food, thus the KCalorie value of a particular serving will vary around that average.

Approximate Composition

An alternative method of estimating the energy value of a food is by calculating the KCalories contributed by the Carbohydrate, Fat, and Protein content as listed in food tables. These calculations are based on the KCalorie value per gram of each of the Energy-yielding Macronutrients, values known as their **fuel factors**.

Note that 1 gram of Fat contains more than twice the number of KCalories as 1 gram of Carbohydrate or Protein. The fuel factor for Alcohol (7 kcal/gram) falls midway between Fat and that of Carbohydrate and Protein.

Using the method of approximate composition, a food containing 12 grams of Carbohydrate, 8 grams of Protein, and 5 grams of Fat would contain 125 kcal.

$$1 \text{ calorie} = 4.1868 \text{ joules}$$
$$1 \text{ BTU} = 1055.056 \text{ joules}$$

FUEL FACTORS

ENERGY SOURCE KCALORIES PER GRAM

Carbohydrate	4
Protein	4
Fat	9
Alcohol	7

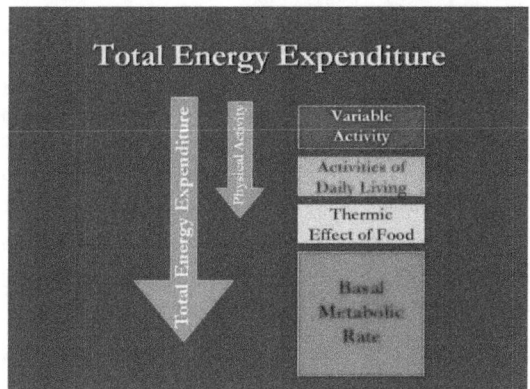

Total Energy Requirement

The total energy expended by an individual stems from three Energy needs: (1) Basal Metabolism, (2) food intake effect, and (3) physical activity. Physical size and **Body Composition**, as well as level of physical activity, influence the Energy needs of a given individual.

Energy expenditure

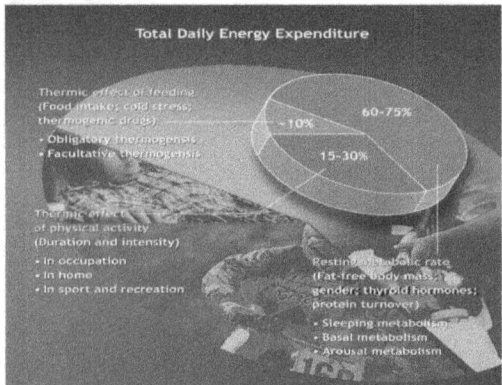

The total amount of Energy used by the body each day is called Total Energy Expenditure.

It includes the Energy needed to maintain basic body functions as well as that needed to fuel physical activity and process food.

In individuals who are growing or pregnant, total energy expenditure also includes the Energy used to deposit new tissues. In women who are Lactating, it includes the Energy used to produce milk. A small amount of Energy is also used to maintain our Body Temperature in a cold environment.

Energy Expenditure for Various Activities

	Calories per Hour (by body weight)				
Type of Activity	100 lb	120 lb	150 lb	180 lb	200 lb
Aerobics (heavy)	363	435	544	653	726
Aerobics (medium)	227	272	340	408	454
Aerobics (light)	136	163	204	245	272
Archery	159	190	238	286	317
Backpacking	408	490	612	735	816

Type of Activity	Calories per Hour (by body weight)				
	100 lb	120 lb	150 lb	180 lb	200 lb
Badminton (doubles)	181	218	272	327	363
Badminton (singles)	231	278	347	416	463
Basketball (nonvigorous)	431	517	646	776	862
Basketball (vigorous)	499	599	748	898	998
Bicycling (6 mph)	159	190	238	286	317
Bicycling (10 mph)	249	299	374	449	499
Bicycling (11 mph)	295	354	442	531	590
Bicycling (12 mph)	340	408	510	612	680
Bicycling (13 mph)	385	463	578	694	771
Billiards	91	109	136	163	181
Bowling	177	212	265	318	354
Boxing—competition	603	724	905	1086	1206
Boxing—sparring	376	452	565	678	753
Calisthenics (heavy)	363	435	544	653	726
Calisthenics (light)	181	218	272	327	363
Canoeing (2.5 mph)	150	180	224	269	299
Canoeing (5 mph)	340	408	510	612	680
Carpentry	227	272	340	408	454
Climbing (mountain)	454	544	680	816	907
Disco dancing	272	327	408	490	544

Type of Activity	Calories per Hour (by body weight)				
	100 lb	120 lb	150 lb	180 lb	200 lb
Ditch digging (hand)	263	316	395	473	526
Fencing	340	408	510	612	680
Fishing (bank/boat)	159	190	238	286	317
Fishing (in waders)	249	299	374	449	499
Football (touch)	340	408	510	612	680
Gardening	145	174	218	261	290
Golf (carry clubs)	227	272	340	408	454
Golf (pull cart)	163	196	245	294	327
Golf (ride in cart)	113	136	170	204	227
Handball (vigorous)	454	544	680	816	907
Hiking (X-country)	249	299	374	449	499
Hiking (mountain)	340	408	510	612	680
Horseback trotting	231	278	347	416	463
Housework	181	218	272	327	363
Hunting (carry load)	272	327	408	490	544
Ice hockey (vigorous)	454	544	680	816	907
Ice skating (10 mph)	263	316	395	473	526
Jazzercise (heavy)	363	435	544	653	726
Jazzercise (medium)	227	272	340	408	454
Jazzercise (light)	136	163	204	245	272

Type of Activity	Calories per Hour (by body weight)				
	100 lb	120 lb	150 lb	180 lb	200 lb
Jog (9 min/mile)	499	599	748	898	998
Jog (10 min/mile)	454	544	680	816	907
Jog (12 min/mile)	385	463	578	694	771
Jog (13 min/mile)	317	381	476	571	635
Jog (14 min/mile)	272	327	408	490	544
Jog (15 min/mile)	227	272	340	408	454
Jog (17 min/mile)	181	218	272	327	363
Lawn mowing (hand)	295	354	442	531	590
Lawn mowing (power)	163	196	245	294	327
Musical instrument playing	113	136	170	204	227
Racquetball (social)	385	463	578	694	771
Racquetball (vigorous)	454	544	680	816	907
Roller skating	231	278	347	416	463
Rowboating (2.5 mph)	200	239	299	359	399
Rowing (11 mph)	590	707	884	1061	1179
Run (5 min/mile)	816	980	1224	1469	1633
Run (6 min/mile)	703	844	1054	1265	1406
Run (7 min/mile)	612	735	918	1102	1224
Run (8 min/mile)	544	653	816	980	1088
Sailing	159	190	238	286	317

Type of Activity	Calories per Hour (by body weight)				
	100 lb	120 lb	150 lb	180 lb	200 lb
Shuffleboard/skeet	136	163	204	245	272
Skiing (X-country)	454	544	680	816	907
Skiing (downhill)	363	435	544	653	726
Square dancing	272	327	407	490	544
Swimming (competitive)	680	816	1020	1224	1361
Swimming (fast)	426	512	639	767	853
Swimming (slow)	349	419	524	629	698
Table tennis	236	283	354	424	472
Tennis (doubles)	227	272	340	408	454
Tennis (singles)	295	354	442	531	590
Tennis (vigorous)	385	463	578	694	771
Volleyball	231	278	347	416	463
Walking (20 min/mile)	159	190	238	286	317
Walking (26 min/mile)	136	163	204	245	272
Water skiing	317	381	476	571	635
Weight lifting (heavy)	408	490	612	735	816
Weight lifting (light)	181	218	272	327	363
Wood chopping (sawing)	295	354	442	531	590

For most people, about 60 to 75% of total energy expenditure is used for **Basal Metabolism.**

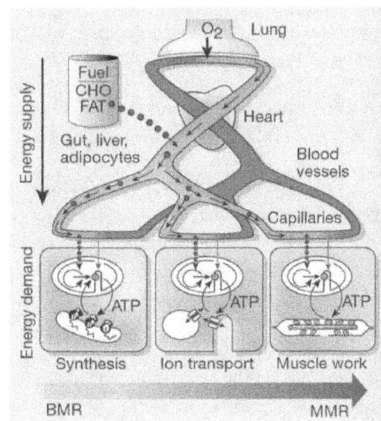

Basal Metabolism includes all the essential metabolic reactions and life-sustaining functions needed to keep you alive, such as breathing, circulating blood, regulating body temperature, synthesizing tissues, removing waste products, and sending nerve signals.

The rate at which energy is used for these basic functions is the **Basal Metabolic Rate (BMR)**. The Energy expended for Basal Metabolism does *not* include the Energy needed for physical activity or for the digestion of food and absorption of Nutrients.

Basal Metabolism is the Energy expended to maintain an awake, resting body that is not digesting food.

Basal Metabolic Rate (BMR) The rate of energy expenditure under resting conditions. It is measured after 12 hours without food or exercise.

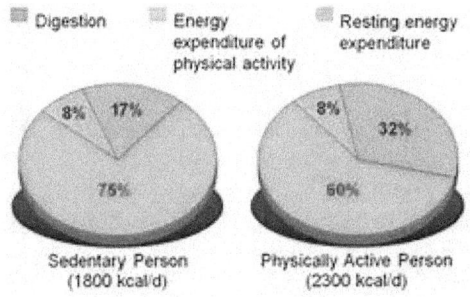

Sedentary Person
(1800 kcal/d)

Physically Active Person
(2300 kcal/d)

BMR increases with increasing body weight and is affected by body composition because it takes more energy to maintain lean tissue than to maintain body Fat.

BMR is generally higher in men than in women because men have a greater amount of lean body mass.

BMR decreases with age, partly because of the decrease in lean body mass that occurs as we get older. BMR is also lower when Calorie intake is consistently below the body's needs. This drop in BMR reduces the amount of Energy needed to maintain body weight.

It is a beneficial adaptation in someone who is starving, but in someone who is trying to lose weight, it is frustrating because it makes weight loss more difficult.

Physical activity is the second major component of total energy expenditure. In most people, physical activity accounts for a smaller proportion of Total Energy Expenditure than Basal Metabolism does—about 15 to 30% of Energy requirements.

The Energy we expend in physical activity includes both planned exercise and daily activities such as walking to work, typing, performing yard work, work-related activities, and even fidgeting.

This ***Non-Exercise Activity Thermogenesis*** (NEAT) includes the Energy expended for everything that is not sleeping, eating, or sports-like exercise. In most people it accounts for the majority of the energy expended for activity and varies enormously, depending on an individual's occupation and daily movements.

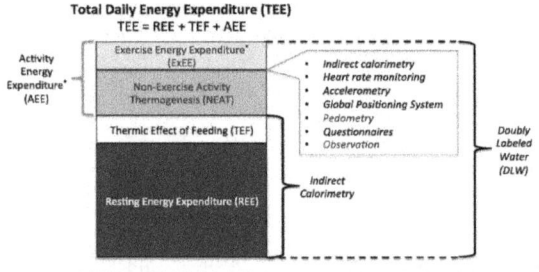

The amount of Energy used for activity depends on the size of the person, how strenuous the activity is, and the length of time it is performed. Because it takes more Energy to move a heavier object, the amount of Energy expended for many activities increases as body weight increases.

More strenuous activities, such as jogging, use more energy than do less strenuous activities, such as walking, but if you walk for an hour, you will probably burn as many calories as you would by jogging for 30 minutes.

We also use energy to digest food and to absorb, metabolize, and store the nutrients from this food.

Table 1	
Thermic Effect of Food	
• Protein	20-30% of calories ingested
• Carbohydrate	5-10% of calories ingested*
• Fats	3-7% of calories ingested

* When carbs are converted to fat (lipogenesis) it requires ~20% of the calories.

The energy used for these processes is called either the **thermic effect of food (TEF)** or diet-induced thermogenesis. This Energy expenditure causes the body temperature to rise slightly for several hours after a person has eaten.

The energy required for TEF is estimated to be about 10% of Energy intake but can vary, depending on the amounts and types of Nutrients consumed

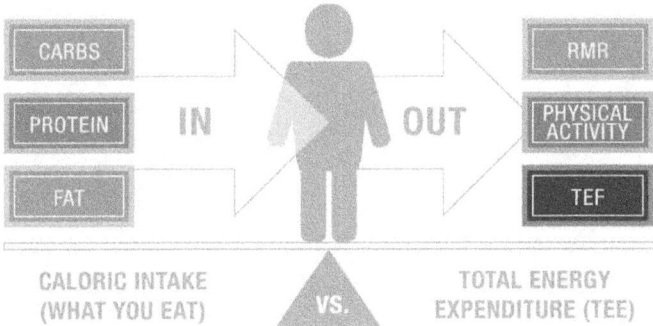

HOW TO CALCULATE YOUR CALORIES

Basal Metabolic Rate (BMR) is the number of calories you would burn with NO activity.

MEN
BMR = 66 +
(6.23 x *weight in lbs*) +
(12.7 x height in inches)
- (6.8 x age)

WOMEN
BMR = 655 +
(4.35 x *weight in lbs*) +
(4.7 x height in inches)
- (4.7 x age)

*(TIP: use **Lean Body weight** (% body fat x weight in lbs) if possible)*

YOUR TARGET DAILY CALORIE NEEDS

1. Little or no exercise: BMR x 1.2

2. Light Exercise/sports 1-3 days/week: BMR x 1.375

3. Medium Exercise/sports 3-5 days/week: BMR x 1.55

4. Hard Exercise/sports 6-7 days a week: BMR x 1.725

5. Intense exercise/sports, physical job or twice/day training): BMR x 1.9

Physical Quantity	Name	Symbol	SI Unit
Force	Newton	N	$kg \bullet m/s^2$
Energy	Joule	J	$kg \bullet m^2/s^2$
Power	Watt	W	$kg \bullet m^2/s^3$

*****

Chapter Fifteen .... SCIENTIFICALLY SPEAKING

*****

At this moment, trillions of Cells in your body are hard at work turning the Chemical Energy of the food you ate yesterday into the Chemical Energy that will keep you alive today.

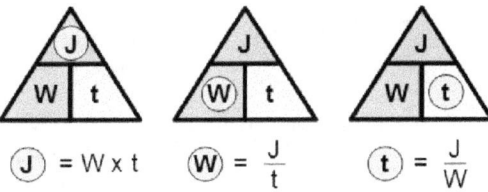

Energy in our Atmosphere generates sweeping winds and powerful storms, while the ocean's Energy drives mighty currents and incessant tides.

Meanwhile, deep within Earth, Energy in the form of Heat is moving the continent on which you are standing.

All situations where energy is expended have one thing in common. If you look at the event closely enough, you will find that, in accord with Newton's laws of Motion, a Force is being exerted on an object to make it move.

When your car burns gasoline, the fuel's energy ultimately turns the wheels of your car, which then exert a force on the road; the road exerts an equal and opposite force on the car, pushing it for- ward.

When you climb the stairs, your muscles exert a force that lifts you upward against gravity. Even in your body's cells, a force is exerted on molecules in chemical reactions.

Energy thus is intimately connected with the application of a force.

$$J = W \times t \qquad W = \frac{J}{t} \qquad t = \frac{J}{W}$$

Work

Scientists say that work is done whenever a force is exerted over a distance. Pick up this book and raise it a foot. Your Muscles applied a Force equal to the weight of the book over a distance of a foot. You did work.

Work = force • distance

This definition of work differs considerably from everyday usage. From a physicist's point of view, if you accidentally drive into a tree and smash your fender, work has been done because a force deformed the car's metal a measurable distance. On the other hand, a physicist would say that you haven't done any work if you spend an hour in a futile effort to move a large boulder, no matter how tired you get. Even though you have exerted a considerable Force, the distance over which you exerted it is negligible.

Physicists provide an exact mathematical definition of their notion of work.

In words: **Work is equal to the Force that is exerted times the Distance over which it is exerted.**

In equation form:

Work = Force x Distance

$$W = F.d$$

In practical terms, even a small force can do a lot of work if it is exerted over a long distance.

As you might expect from this equation, units of work are equal to a force unit times a distance unit. In the metric system of units, where force is measured in new- tons (abbreviated N), work is measured in newton-meters (N-m). For reference, a newton is roughly equal to the force exerted on your hand by a baseball (or by seven Fig Newtons!).

Joules

$$\text{Force} = \text{mass} * \text{acceleration}$$

$$\text{Force} = kg \cdot m/s^2$$

$$1 \text{ Newton} = 1 kg \cdot m/s^2 = \text{a measure of force}$$

$$\text{Therefore, } 1 \text{ Joule} = 1 \text{ Newton} \cdot m$$

This unit is given the special name joule, after the English scientist James Prescott Joule (1818–1889), one of the first people to understand the properties of energy. One joule is defined as the amount of work done when a force of one newton is exerted over a distance of one meter.

In the English system of units, where force is measured in pounds, work is measured in a unit called the foot-pound (usually abbreviated ft-lb).

Energy

Energy is defined as the ability to do work. If a system is capable of exerting a force over a distance, then that system possesses energy. The amount of a system's energy, which can be recorded in joules or foot-pounds (the same units used for work), is a measure of how much work the system might do. When a system runs out of energy, it simply can't do any more work.

ATP and Energy

- Releasing Energy
  - Energy stored in ATP is released by breaking the chemical bond between the second and third phosphates.

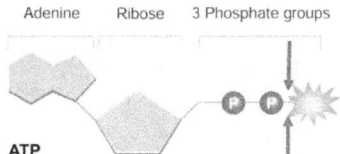

Power

Power provides a measure of both the amount of work done (or, equivalently, the amount of energy expended) and the time it takes to do that work. In order to complete a physi- cal task quickly, you must generate more power than if you do the same task slowly.

If you run up a flight of stairs, your muscles need to generate more power than they would if you walked up the same flight, even though you expend the same amount of energy in either case. A power hitter in baseball swings the bat faster, converting the chemical energy in his muscles to kinetic energy more quickly than most other players

Scientists define power as the rate at which work is done, or the rate at which energy is expended.

In words: Power is the amount of work done divided by the time it takes to do that work.

$$\text{Power} = \frac{\text{work}}{\text{time}}$$

If you do more Work in a given span of time, or do a task in a shorter time, you use more Power. In the metric system, power is measured in watts after James Watt (1736-1819), the Scottish inventor who developed the modern steam engine that powered the Industrial Revolution (Figure 3-4). The Watt, a unit of measurement that you probably encounter every day, is defined as the expenditure of 1 Joule of Energy in 1 second:

The unit of 1,000 watts (corresponding to an expenditure of 1,000 joules per second) is called a Kilowatt and is a commonly used measurement of Electrical Power. The English system, on the other hand, uses the more colorful unit horsepower, which is defined as 550 foot-pounds per second.

The familiar rating of a lightbulb (60 watts or 100 watts, for example) is a measure of the rate of energy that the lightbulb consumes when it is operating. As another familiar example, most electric hand tools or appliances in your home will be labeled with a power rating in watts.

The equation we have introduced defining power as energy divided by time may be rewritten as follows:

energy (joules)   power (watts)   time (seconds)

This important equation allows you (and the electric company) to calculate how much energy you consume (and how much you have to pay for). Note from this equation that, although the joule is the standard scientific unit for energy, energy can also be measured in units of power   time, such as the familiar kilowatt-hour (often abbreviated kWh) that appears on your electric bill.

*****

Conclusion

*****

We are created in a Magnificently Perfect vehicle/body to make manifest from within self the Highest Expression of Humanity = the GOD....Whose Image and Likeness we are Created In. The Mind, Body and Spirit are intricately connected, what Effects one – Effects ALL.

*A physical ailment causes mental distress and stress, which in-turn manifests in us having a 'low' Spirit/Emotios (Moody, Sad, Easily Upset).

*Thoughts/Emotions (Positive/Negative) produce corresponding Hormones that CHANGE our physical Body INTO that Thought/Emotion.

*Mental Stress and Distress causes production/release of low Energy Hormones, which in-turn causes a physical ailment/reaction, which in-turn manifests a Low/Bad Spirit/Emotional state and temperament.

* Low/Bad Spirit/Emotions causes corresponding low-energy Thoughts to be produced, which in-turn produces/releases low-energy Hormones, which in-turn manifests as a physical ailment.

The food we chose for Nutrition/Energy plays a vital role in the above equation because Nutrition/Energy not only fuels and help us grow, our Brain is Glucose dependent, and eating our favorite food always makes us Feel Good!!!

We must understand that Nutrition is personal, and that even though common foods can be shared, the amount varies to the specific individual. This amount is predicated by the amount of Energy expended for which we need to replace.

If we performed little to no activity (sedentary), then we should consume the equivalent in Nutrition/Energy = with attention to consume NO MORE THAN NEEDED!

Once we can change the Understanding of food from a culinary/taste perspective and focus on food being Energy, we will make better food choices = Decrease in pre-mature death = Increase in Life-span !!

In fact, our Nutritional/Energy needs have to be switched from 'Eating' to other forms of Energy Extraction.

NEW PARADIGMS ON HOW TO EAT TO LIVE !!!!

We come from the Earth and ALL our Solutions are found IN the Earth.......ALL we have to do is turn back to the Earth and Extract what we Need !!!!

Every part of us is related to the Earth....Our Skin is like the Leaves/Skin of the Plants......Our Blood is as the Water on the Earth.......Our Bones is as the Rocks on the Earth..

The SAME Chemical Action (Photosynthesis) that allows the Leaves of the Plants to transform the Un-Seen Life Energy of the Sun into a Seen Chemical Compound happens with our SKIN....

Allowing the Melanocytes in the Epidermis to Absorb the Un-Seen Life Energy of the Sun into Melanin, Vitamin D and other forms of Energy.

We 'Eat' or Extract the same Nutrients/Energy without the unnecessary wear and tear on our Digestive System.

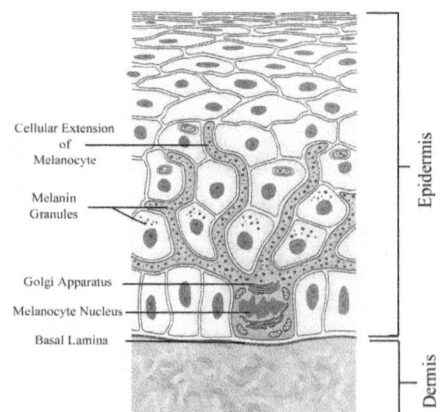

EATING TO LIVE !!!!

The Roots of Plants have the Primary function of Extracting the Un-Seen Life Energy from the Earth, so that they Plant can transform it into a Seen Chemical Element, making a perfect vehicle for us to Extract and Harvest the Life Energy that we need to replenish and maintain self.

The Roots of Plants are perfectly constructed to Seek and Extract the Life Energy deep within the Earth. Our Legs are similar to the Roots of Plants. When two Objects of Mass touch = Exchange of Electrons/Energy.

When we Stand and ROOT ourselves IN the Earth, Barefoot, our Feet become like the Roots of Plants and Extract the Life Energy from the Earth = 'Eating' or Extracting Nutrients/Energy without wear and tear on our Digestive System.

Nutrition should be viewed from the perspective of utilizing the BEST method for us to Extract the Life Energy from the Sun and Earth!

The Best method is NOT through 'Eating'. If we aren't growing our own food, then we can almost be assured in consuming nutritionally deficient foods. Grocery stores have to have their produce shipped BEFORE it has naturally ripened to ensure that it doesn't 'Rot' on route. With the influx of government mandated GMO crops, we literally DON'T KNOW WHAT WE ARE EATING.

The Best way for us to 'Eat' or Extract the Nutrients/Energy is by Naturally Absorbing the Sun with our Skin (Sun-bathing) and Rooting Self IN the Earth(Grounding) and extracting the Energy through the Exchange of Electrons.

Achieving and Maintaining Supreme Health and Fitness by Increasing the level of Knowledge and Science of Life!!

PEACE

Sean Ali, BS Health and Wellness

*Supreme Health and Fitness

*****

Facts & Figures

*****

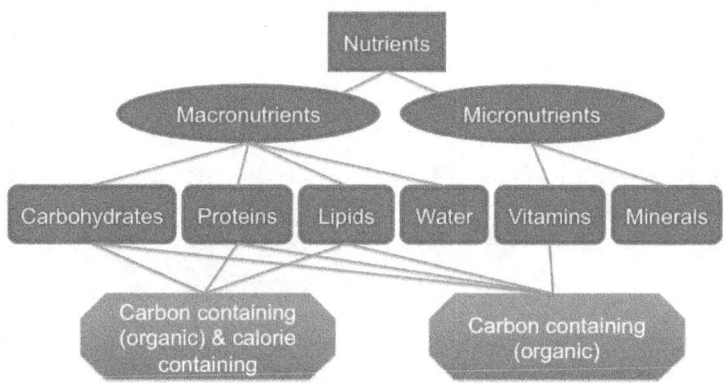

Energy transformations in the human body are accompanied with continuous production of heat

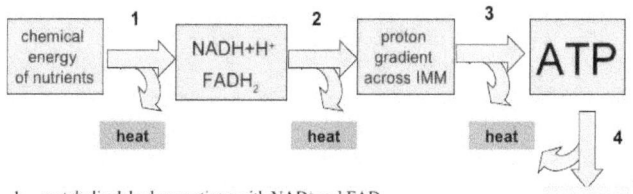

1 ... metabolic dehydrogenations with NAD^+ and FAD

2 ... respiratory chain (oxidation of reduced cofactors + reduction of O_2 to H_2O)

3 ... oxidative phosphorylation, IMM inner mitochondrial membrane

4 ... transformation of chemical energy of ATP into work + some heat

 ... high energy systems   4

INSULIN'S ROLE IN BODY AND BRAIN

Insulin, long recognized as a primary regulator of blood glucose, is now also understood to play key roles in neuroplasticity, neuromodulation, and neurotrophism, the process of neuronal growth, stimulated by neuronal differentiation and survival.

NEUROLOGIC INFLUENCE

Insulin activates insulin receptors and downstream signaling molecules in the brain and spinal cord, as well as insulin-sensitive glucose transporters in the peripheral insulin-sensitive tissues (liver, muscle, fat). Through these mechanisms, insulin participates in feeding behavior, reward pathways, whole body metabolism, and normal emotional and cognitive brain functions. The dysregulation of insulin-mediated signaling pathways in the brain is implicated in neurodegenerative diseases such as Alzheimer's and psychiatric disorders such as schizophrenia.

High blood glucose

Raises blood sugar

Glucagon stimulates the conversion of stored glycogen in the liver into glucose

Glucagon released by alpha cells of pancreas

Glycogen

Glucose

Insulin stimulates the liver to remove glucose from the blood and stores it as glycogen.

Insulin released by beta cells of pancreas

Tissue cells take up glucose from blood.

Lowers blood sugar

Low blood glucose

Insulin can cross the blood-brain barrier.

Cortex

Hypothalamus

Midbrain

METABOLIC INFLUENCE

Insulin is one of the primary hormones involved in blood glucose regulation. Its dysregulation is associated with obesity and diabetes.

Insulin receptors are expressed throughout the brain, including the midbrain, the hypothalamus, and the cortex.

Human Energy Systems

Anaerobic
1-10 sec   ATP-CP   ATP & Phosphocreatine
30-120 sec   Lactic Acid   Carbohydrate

Aerobic   (Oxidative)
>5 minutes   Carbohydrate and Fat
- Moderate-High Intensity   75% Carb / 25% fat
- Moderate Intensity   50% carb/ 50% fat
- Lower Intensity or >High Duration   >Fat contribution
- Resting   80%-90% Fat

Where Food Scientists Work

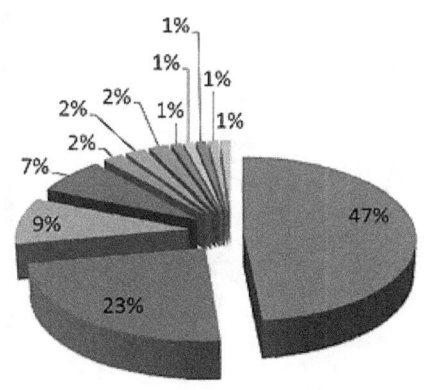

- Food/beverage processor
- Ingredient manufacturer/supplier
- Academia
- Other
- Foodservice
- Food retailer
- Government
- Processing equipment manufacturer/supplier
- Scientific/trade organization
- Testing laboratory
- Private research facility
- Packaging manufacturer/supplier

THE THREE
UNHEALTHY WHITES

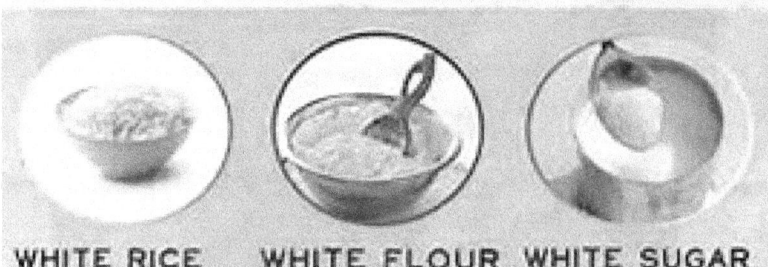

WHITE RICE   WHITE FLOUR WHITE SUGAR

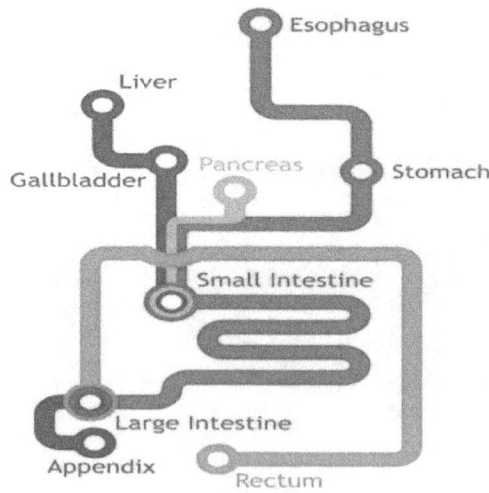

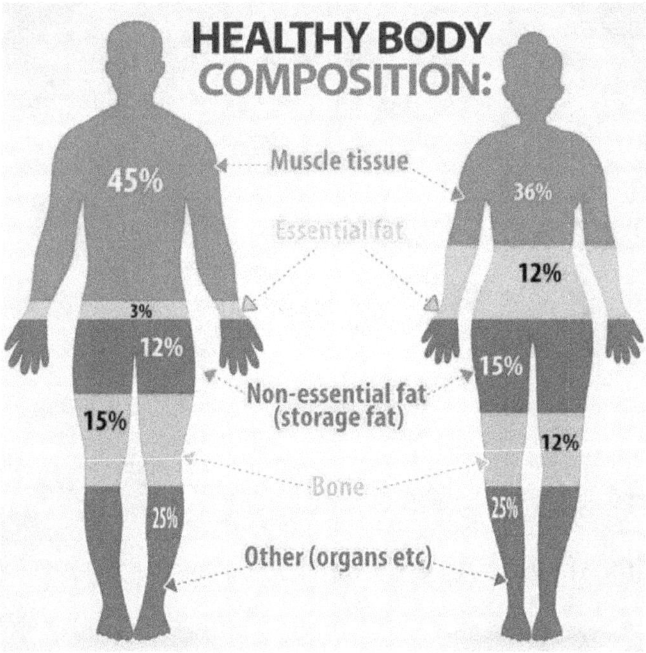
HEALTHY BODY
COMPOSITION:
Muscle tissue
45%
36%
Essential fat
12%
3%
12%
15%
Non-essential fat
(storage fat)
15%
12%
Bone
25%
25%
Other (organs etc)

IS THAT REALLY IN MY MEAT?

ANTIBIOTIC-RESISTANT BACTERIA CONTAMINATION

SALMONELLA & CAMPYLOBACTER BACTERIA FOUND IN...

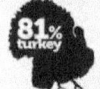 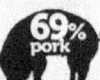 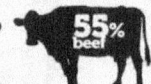

81% turkey   **69%** pork   **55%** beef   **39%** chicken

Salmonella and Campylobacter bacteria cause **millions** of cases of food poisoning a year.

Of the **chicken** tested, **53%** was **tainted** with an **antibiotic-resistant form of E.coli.**

Certain strains of E.coli cause urinary tract infections, pneumonia and other illnesses.

29.9 million pounds of antibiotics were sold in 2011 for meat and poultry production, *compared to*

7.7 million pounds sold for human use

References:

*****

Cook, JT, Frank, DA, Levenson, SM, et al. Child food insecurity increases risks posed by household food insecurity to young children's health. *J Nutr.* 2006; 136:1073.

American Dietetic Association. Position of the American Dietetic Association: food insecurity in the United States. *J Am Diet Assoc.* 2010; 110:1368.

Robaina, KA, Martin, KS. Food insecurity, poor diet quality and obesity among food pantry participants in Hartford, CT. *J Nutr Educ Behav.* 2012; 45(2):159.

Gany, F, Bari, S, Crist, M, et al. Food insecurity: limitations of emergency food resources for our patients. *J Urban Health.* 2013; 90(3):552.

Morley, JE, Thomas, DR, Wilson, MM. Cachexia: pathophysiology and clinical relevance. *Am J Clin Nutr.* 2006; 83:735.

Richard, C, Couture, P, Desroches, S, et al. Effect of the Mediterranean diet with or without weight loss on markers of inflammation in men with metabolic syndrome. *Obesity.* 2013; 21(1):51.

Schlenker, Eleanor, Joyce Gilbert. *Williams' Essentials of Nutrition and Diet Therapy, 11th Edition.* Mosby, 102014. VitalBook file.

Trefil, James. *The Sciences: An Integrated Approach, 7th Edition.* Wiley, 09/2012. VitalBook file.

Thygerson, Alton L. *Fit to Be Well: Essential Concepts, 3rd Edition.* Jones & Bartlett Learning, 20120213. VitalBook file.

U.S. Department of Health and Human Services, Public Health Service, *The Surgeon General's report on nutrition and health* PHS Publication No. 88-50210. U.S. Government Printing Office, Washington, D.C., 1988.

Food and Nutrition Board, Institute of Medicine. *Diet and health: implications for reducing chronic disease risk.* Washington, D.C.: National Academies Press; 1989.

U.S. Department of Health and Human Services, *Healthy People 2010: Final review.* National Center for Health Statistics, Centers for Disease Control and Prevention, Washington, D.C., 2011. at. http://www.cdc.gov/nchs/healthy_people/hp2010/hp2010_final_review.htm/ [Accessed on July 16, 2012].

U.S. Department of Health and Human Services, *Healthy People 2020: 2020 Topics and Objectives.* U.S. Department of Health and Human Services, Washington, D.C., 2013. at. http://www.healthypeople.gov/2020/default.aspx [Accessed on August 19, 2013].

Further Readings and Resources:

Academy of Nutrition and Dietetics. Position of the Academy of Nutrition and Dietetics: total diet approach to healthy eating. *J Acad Nutr Diet*. 2013; 113:307.

[This review helps us understand the importance of the overall food pattern, not just one day or one meal.]

Klurfeld, DM. What do government agencies consider in the debate over added sugars? *Adv Nutr*. 2013; 4(2):257.

[Dr. Klurfeld reviews the trends in added sugar intake and the health implications for the American public.]

25 Reilly, PR, DeBusk, RM. Ethical and legal issues in nutritional genomics. *J Am Diet Assoc*. 2008; 108:36.

[When it becomes possible to customize nutrition intervention based on an individual's genetic code, there are various issues that will need to be considered.]

Slavin, J. Dietary Guidelines. Are we on the right path? *Nutr Today*. 2012; 47(5):245.

[This nutrition expert raises questions about the 2010 Dietary Guidelines and provides suggestions for change when the 2015 Guidelines are developed.]

U.S. Department of Agriculture, Center for Nutrition Policy and Promotion, *An evidence-based approach to reviewing the science on nutrition and health, Nutrition Insight 38*. U.S. Government Printing Office, Alexandria, Va., 2008. from. http://www.cnpp.usda.gov/Publications/NutritionInsights/Insight38.pdf [Retrieved on August 19, 2013].

[This publication provides a helpful summary on why we need to apply an evidence-based approach to our practice and gives an example of the process.]

U.S. Department of Agriculture, Center for Nutrition Policy and Promotion, *The Food Environment, Eating Out, and Body Weight: A Review of the Evidence, Nutrition Insight 49*. U.S. Government Printing Office, Alexandria, Va., 2012. from. http://www.cnpp.usda.gov/Publications/NutritionInsights/Insight49.pdf [Retrieved on August 19, 2013].

[This review cites evidence from the Nutrition Evidence Library (NEL) linking frequency of meals away from home and risk of overweight, and helps us understand why this occurs.]

Wellman, NS, Borra, ST, Schleman, JC, et al. Trends in news media reporting of food and health issues. *Nutr Today*. 2011; 46(3):123. [May-June].

Websites of Interest:

• U.S. Department of Agriculture: Nutrition Evidence Library, 2013. This website provided the scientific evidence reviewed by the 2010 Dietary Guidelines Advisory Committee in preparation of their report. http://www.cnpp.usda.gov/NEL.htm.

• U.S. Department of Health and Human Services, 2008. *Physical Activity Guidelines for Americans.* This Web site presents science-based physical activity guidelines for both youth and adults along with educational materials for health professionals and consumers. http://www.health.gov/paguidelines/guidelines/default.aspx.

• U.S. Department of Agriculture, Food Surveys Research Group: *What We Eat in America: Data from the National Health and Nutrition Examination Survey.* This site describes the food and nutrient intakes of Americans according to age, sex, race, ethnicity, and economic status. www.ars.usda.gov/Services/docs.htm?docid=15044.

• U.S. Department of Health and Human Services, National Heart, Lung and Blood Institute: *Keep an Eye on Portion Distortion.* This site describes portion sizes and how they have changed over the years. http://hp2010.nhlbihin.net/portion/keep.htm.

OxyGen: The Breath Of LIFE In Atomic Form
Authored by Sean Ali

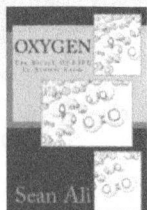

List Price: **$30.00**

6" x 9" (15.24 x 22.86 cm)
Full Color on White paper
134 pages

ISBN-13: **978-1541272170** (CreateSpace-Assigned)
ISBN-10: **154127217X**
BISAC: Health & Fitness / Healthy Living

Peace and Blessings of Health!

*Do YOU have health issues that YOU want to over-come?
*Do YOU want to Improve the Quality of YOUR Life?
*Do YOU want to achieve ABUNDANT LIFE?
*** THEN THIS BOOK IS FOR YOU!! ***

Oxygen IS the Breath Of LIFE in Atomic form!

This short work is a composition of Scientific, Medical and Spiritually based research , compiled into a comprehensive, easily read and understood format, designed to Help the reader achieve and maintain their own Supreme Health and Fitness!

We have 3 major functions - Eating, Drinking and Breathing, that must be performed in order for us to be considered Alive......... Of these 3 functions, Breathing is the least explored, taught or performed properly - BUT THE MOST IMPORTANT.

We can go 7-10 days without Food before signs of Nutritional deficiency. We can go 3-7 days without Water before we present symptoms........ But, 1 Minute of Oxygen deprivation/deficiency causes Cellular Damage!

Our Cells need 2 elements for Growth and Reproduction = OXYGEN & GLUCOSE !

Let's explore and discover the Amazing Power of Oxygen and the Natural Ability to Heal Self!

OXYGEN IS THE BREATH OF LIFE IN ATOMIC FORM !

OPEN THIS BOOK - and take the steps to Successfully Build Your own Supreme Health & Fitness!

PEACE!

LIFE Energy: The Sun, Glucose & WHY Humans Are Herbivores!
Authored by Sean Ali

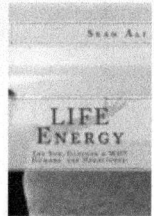

List Price: **$30.00**

6" x 9" (15.24 x 22.86 cm)
Full Color on White paper
156 pages

ISBN-13: **978-1544622842** (CreateSpace-Assigned)
ISBN-10: **1544622848**
BISAC: Medical / Diet Therapy

Peace and Blessings of Health!

*Do YOU have a health issue that YOU would like to over-come?
*Do YOU want to Improve the Quality of YOUR Life?
*Do YOU want to experience ABUNDANT LIFE?

*** OPEN THIS BOOK - NOW!!! ***

This small book is written with the purpose of re-examining the role of Nutrition in health care and everyday Life.....LIFE IS ENERGY.....Nutrition is a descriptive term to describe how we replenish our Life Energy.
Understanding Nutrition is the equivalent of understanding Energy
Knowledge of Nutrition enables us to make precise Energy adjustments through Nutrients to provide the proper Energy needed for all our body functions/tasks – from achieving Homeostasis, facilitating our Growth, Development and Self-Healing.
We come from the Earth and all our Solutions are manifested from the Earth...... All we have to do is return back to the Earth and extract what we need.
Food is our naturally occurring vehicle, perfectly designed for administering the Life Energy in the form of Nutrition.
Our Food choices and the Energy released from it, presents as either the root cause of our dis-ease or the base for our Solution.
From our Cells to our Immune system, we are Created to Heal and Regenerate Self with the aide of proper Nutrition/Energy.
Our Food is our Medicine ONLY with proper application...... There is no in-between, which means that we are either eating to die – OR – Eating To LIVE !!!
Energy is the Key to LIFE and we Know that the Sun is the Source of all Energy, so if we focus on how to obtain as much Sun in the form of food as possible = the Key to Nutritional Health and Therapy.
Let us explore and examine Life Energy and how to obtain the best Quality and Value so that we may successfully manifest the Best out of Life and Enjoy a long, active and fruitful Life-span!

Achieving and Maintaining Supreme Health and Fitness by increasing the level of Knowledge and Science of Life!

Peace
Sean Ali

Understanding Carbohydrates: LIFE Energy, Fiber, Sugar and Starch!
Authored by Sean Ali

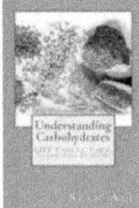

List Price: **$27.00**

6" x 9" (15.24 x 22.86 cm)
Full Color on White paper
140 pages

ISBN-13: **978-1543023763** (CreateSpace-Assigned)
ISBN-10: **1543023762**
BISAC: Health & Fitness / Healthy Living

Peace and Blessings of Health!

"Do YOU have health issues that YOU want to over-come?
"Do YOU want to Improve the Quality of YOUR Life?
"Do YOU want to experience ABUNDANT LIFE?

"** THEN THIS BOOK IS FOR YOU!! ***

There is a disproportionate amount of fad diets and food-like TOXIC items that are available and which we are bombarded
with that promote a detrimentally 'low' or 'no' Carb meal plan that goes TOTALLY against ALL Nutritional science and
evidence of the function of Carbohydrates.
There is little to no serious governmental regulation of these types of claims or food-like items and most are cases of clever
advertisement vs actual claims of quality and value.
This small book has been produced to provide understanding of the Nutritional and Life value of Carbohydrates - from a
Scientific analogy, while simultaneously shedding light on these false claims and food-like products so that YOU can make
the Best Life choices for YOUR successful Growth & Development!
Let us explore and learn about our Primary Energy source and become able to make the best Nutritional choices.
OPEN THIS BOOK - and Begin the steps to Successfully Build and Maintain Your own Supreme Health and Fitness!

Peace !
Sean Ali

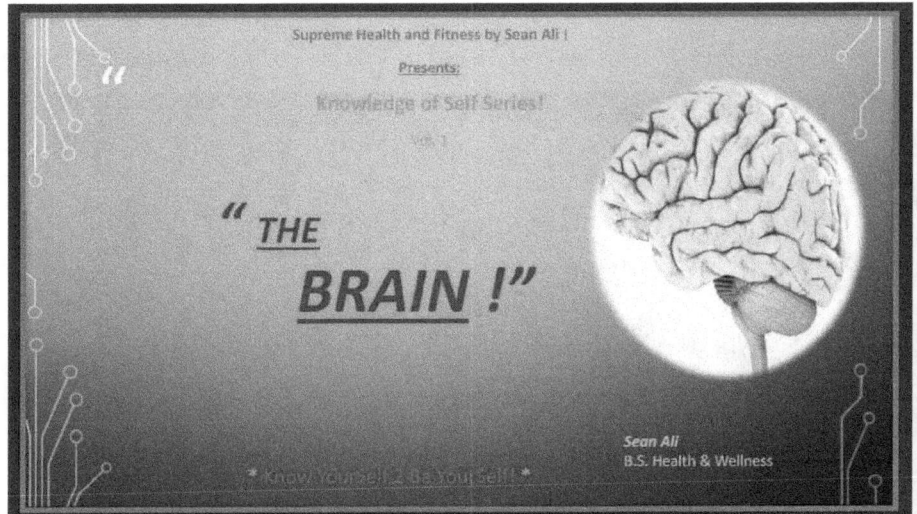

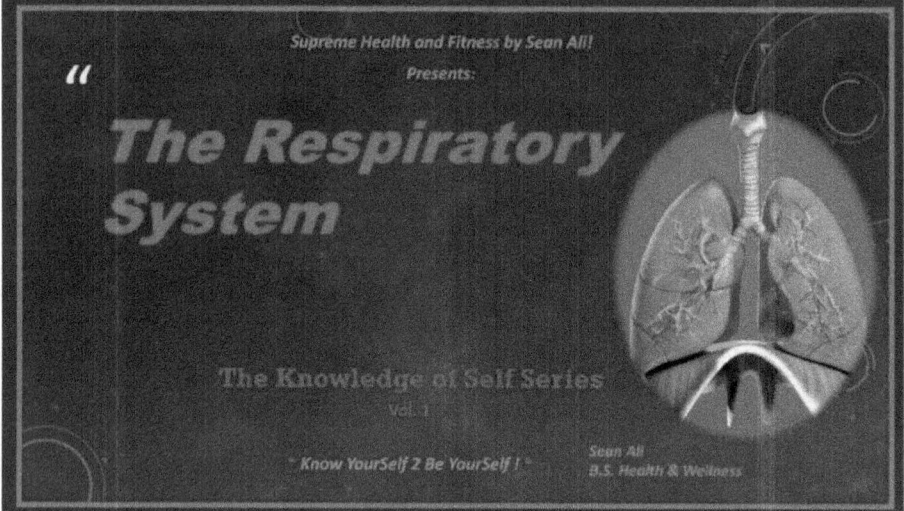

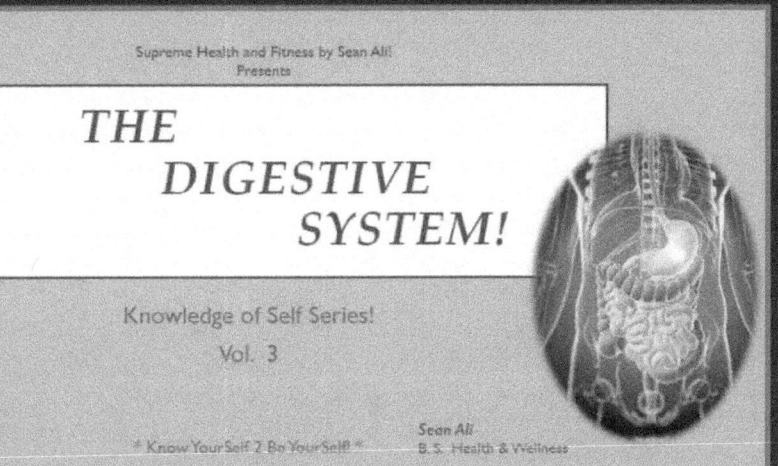

www.ingramcontent.com/pod-product-compliance
Lightning Source LLC
Chambersburg PA
CBHW071716170526
45165CB00005B/2040